Bullying Prevention and Intervention at School

Jacob U'Mofe Gordon
Editor

Bullying Prevention and Intervention at School

Integrating Theory and Research into Best Practices

Springer

Editor
Jacob U'Mofe Gordon
University of Kansas
Lawrence, KS, USA

University of Ghana
Accra, Ghana

ISBN 978-3-030-07033-5 ISBN 978-3-319-95414-1 (eBook)
https://doi.org/10.1007/978-3-319-95414-1

This Springer imprint is published by the registered company Springer Nature Switzerland AG.
The registered company address is: Gewerbestrasse 11, 6330 Cham, Switzerland

Preface

The prevalence of bullying and its negative impact on American society has been well documented in related literature. Millions of children and youth are also victims of bullying throughout the globe. The consequences of bullying may constitute an eminent danger to global peace and security as a health and safety issue. The impact on all segments of the global community, especially around educational settings, undermines human rights and the capacity of the educational sector to train the future leaders. The response to this disturbing phenomenon has been widespread; they have been mostly school-based. These anti-bullying programs are primarily designed to reduce bullying and its related negative impact in the schools. It is important to note that there are about 14,000 school districts in America and about 81.5 million K-12 students with a budget in excess of $500 billion per year. Thus, the reduction and eventual elimination of bullying in American schools poses a tremendous challenge to American society.

The nature of the challenge may be examined from four perspectives: (1) the development of appropriate bullying prevention theories, (2) the policy dimension, (3) program development (prevention, intervention, and recovery), and (4) program evaluation. The response to bullying from anti-bullying community has been multifaceted; they range from school district bullying zero tolerance policy to T-shirts, social and emotional learning (SEL) training, restorative and disciplinary approaches to the most comprehensive Olweus model, and the Friends for Change. Yet research findings indicate the lack of adequate program evaluation to determine the effectiveness of anti-bullying efforts and their cost-effectiveness. Equally important are existing gaps between bullying prevention theories and practices. This book promises to change the situation. It examines emerging theories in bullying continuum of service.

The book has been organized into eight chapters. The first chapter is an in-depth literature review of the current state of bullying. The chapter presents a systematic review of the literature on bullying theories; policies; anti-bullying programs, especially school-based programs; and the state of program monitoring and evaluation. The second chapter examines the predictors of bullying behaviors; using Adlerian theoretical model explains that individuals who engage in social useless behaviors would be more likely to engage in bullying and other negative behaviors. The third chapter explores the application of bibliotherapy as a strategy for advancing the continuum of service in bullying: prevention, intervention, and recovery. Bibliotherapy may be defined as the use of books, literature, and library materials as therapy in the treatment of mental health or psychological disorder. The fourth chapter focuses on the importance of coaching teachers and school administrators on how to detect and intervene in bullying at school settings. The objective is to improve the teacher detection of bullying behaviors. Chapter 5 proposes a promising approach to reduce cyberbullying in youth and society in general. It acknowledges the current lack of empirical data in cyberbullying prevention and intervention; it provides recommendations for moving forward. Chapters 6 and 7 bring an international perspective to focus. Chapter 6 evaluates bullying in secondary schools in Greece. With a collaborative evaluation research between researchers from Greece and Australia, the chapter documents the outcome of an anti-bullying program that places emphasis on the training of students and teachers on bullying coping strategies. Chapter 7 draws on the team work of researchers from the University of Cape Town in South Africa. It examines the impact of mobile bullying in South Africa with a focus on the victims of mobile bullying. It builds on previous research on violence in Southern Africa by the United Nations Educational, Scientific and Cultural Organization (UNESCO). The final chapter is a response to the research findings which document the lack of empirical data on program evaluation. It examines several evaluation models, including the Olweus, the social and emotional learning (SEL), and the ecological approach, and probes the application of the logic model as the most effective tool for conceptualizing, monitoring, and evaluating anti-bullying programs. The chapter concludes with recommended standards for program evaluation and guiding principles for evaluators.

The final word in the chapters is a conclusion drawn from the research findings of each chapter and recommendations for future directions in the anti-bullying enterprise.

Lawrence, KS, USA Jacob U'Mofe Gordon

Acknowledgments

The path to completing this book has been challenging and rewarding in many ways. The journey began in 2015 when I became a member of the Board of Directors of the International Bullying Prevention Association (IBPA). Since my first meeting as a board member and attendance at its Annual International Conference in Denver, Colorado, in 2015, I have been inspired to embark on this journey to produce this volume. My overarching goal is to enhance current anti-bullying theories and illuminate successful and effective practices. Of course, I could not have done it alone. Many professionals who are committed to bullying prevention/intervention/recovery research and practice made significant contributions to the process and to the final outcome.

First, I would like to thank my colleagues on the Board of Directors of the IBPA, especially Executive Director Ms. Lynn Lonsway for the opportunity to learn and to serve on the Board. Second, I would like to acknowledge and thank all of the contributors to this volume for submitting their valuable research in this field. I appreciate their thoughtful consideration of my editorial suggestions. Third, I want to acknowledge the role of Senior Editor, Ms. Judy Jones, for navigating me through the process of publishing this book with Springer. And, finally, I express my appreciation to my wife, Dr. Barbara McDade Gordon, Associate Professor Emerita, University of Florida, for her technical assistance and editorial comments.

Contents

Contributors

Eleni Andreou Department of Primary Education, University of Thessaly, Volos, Greece

Patricia Agatston Prevention/Intervention Center, Cobb County School District, Marietta, GA, USA

Catherine P. Bradshaw Curry School of Education, University of Virginia, Charlottesville, USA

Eleni Didaskalou School of Education, Flinders University, Adelaide, Australia

Reade Dowda Clinical Mental Counseling Program, Fort Hays State University, Hays, KS, USA

Jacob U'Mofe Gordon University of Kansas, Lawrence, KS, USA

University of Ghana, Accra, Ghana

Susan E. Henderson Department of Counselor Education, Sam Houston State University, Huntsville, TX, USA

Stacy R. Johnson Bloomberg School of Public Health, Johns Hopkins University, Baltimore, MD, USA

Michael Kyobe Department of Information Systems, University of Cape Town, Cape Town, South Africa

Kristine E. Larson Bloomberg School of Public Health, Johns Hopkins University, Baltimore, MD, USA

Susan Limber Institute on Family and Neighborhood Life, Psychology Department, Clemson University, Clemson, SC, USA

Shallen Lusinga Department of Information Systems, University of Cape Town, Cape Town, South Africa

Bridgitt L. Mitchell Early Childhood Education, Colorado Community Colleges Online, Colorado Springs, CO, USA

Elise T. Pas Bloomberg School of Public Health, Johns Hopkins University, Baltimore, MD, USA

Stephanie J. Richards Curriculum and Instruction, Tennessee Tech University, Cookeville, TN, USA

Rebecca A. Robles-Piña Department of Counselor Education, Sam Houston State University, Huntsville, TX, USA

Christina Roussi-Vergou University of Thessaly, Volos, Greece

Phillip Slee School of Education, Flinders University, Adelaide, Australia

Grace Skrzypiec School of Education, Flinders University, Adelaide, Australia

Kristen Pennycuff Trent Curriculum and Instruction, Tennessee Tech University, Cookeville, TN, USA

Tracy E. Waasdorp Bloomberg School of Public Health, Johns Hopkins University, Baltimore, MD, USA

About the Editor

Jacob U'Mofe Gordon, PhD is Professor Emeritus at the University of Kansas, Fulbright Program Senior Specialist, and the Kwame Nkrumah Endowed Chair at the University of Ghana, 2012–2015. He is the author and/or coauthor of 26 books, numerous articles in academic journals, book chapters, monographs, and research reports. His diverse academic publications include *Managing Multi-culturalism in Substance Abuse Services* (1994), *A Systems Change Approach to Substance Abuse Prevention* (1997), *The Role of Higher Education in Alcohol and Other Drug Abuse Prevention* (1993), *African Presence in Black America* (2004), and *An Anthology of African Presidential Leadership and Governance* (2017). He is the recipient of many honors and awards and serves on several boards, including the International Bullying Prevention Association (IBPA) and the University of Kansas School of Languages, Literatures and Cultures. He was an international approved evaluator for the Millennium Challenge Corporation (MCC) and served as program evaluator for the Robert Wood Johnson Foundation (RWJF) Fighting Back in Kansas City, Missouri.

Chapter 1
The State of Bullying in Schools

Bridgitt L. Mitchell

Introduction

Bullying is a pervasive social problem within schools that warrants comprehensive solutions. The systemic nature of this epidemic affects not only those who are bullied but also students who bully others and are witnesses to bullying. Blake et al. (2015) argue that "students may assume different yet fluid roles in the bullying continuum that have overlapping effects on the participating youth's psychological functioning" (p. 136). Students may also be subjected to physical harm resulting from bullying behaviors. Therefore, bullying is considered a public health threat that impacts the individual both mentally and physically.

There is also evidence that negative school climates are influenced by families' and education professionals' views, beliefs, and behaviors in regard to bullying (Bradshaw, 2013). The ideology around bullying within the students' primary environments (home and school) drives conflict management, problem-solving, and socio-emotional competency in group settings. Thus, it is beneficial when adults model desired social behaviors and foster environments grounded in trust and mutual respect as well as intervene when inappropriate behaviors occur. As such, many schools have adopted bullying prevention programs and strategies that are specific to the kinds of bullying prevalent in schools. While there is continued support for anti-bullying interventions, it is unclear of the long-term impact of such models.

B. L. Mitchell (✉)
Early Childhood Education, Colorado Community Colleges Online,
Colorado Springs, CO, USA

J. U. Gordon (ed.), *Bullying Prevention and Intervention at School*,
https://doi.org/10.1007/978-3-319-95414-1_1

Definition

Before discussing the incidence of bullying, it is necessary to have a working definition. According to Olweus (1994), bullying is victimization that is characterized by unwanted aggressive behavior, an act repeated over time, and involves an interpersonal relationship that has an imbalance of power. It is important to note that bullying is multidimensional and can include an act traditionally defined as well as those promulgated by societal trends such as social media, i.e., cyberbullying. Further, it is a "pattern of behavior rather than an isolated event, and it has an adverse impact on the victim, bully, and the bystanders" (UNESCO, 2017). Therefore, the impact of bullying manifests across the entire school environment and influences relational norms.

There are two modes of bullying: direct which are aggressive behaviors that occur in the presence of the targeted student and indirect, aggressive behaviors not directly communicated to the targeted student (Gladden, Vivolo-Kantor, Hamburger, & Lumpkin, 2014). These varying modes increase the complexity of bullying in that there is not always a clearly identified way that the behaviors occur to the student. Thus, it is difficult to ascertain effective prevention and intervention strategies.

Gladden et al. (2014) defined the types of bullying as physical, verbal, relational, and damage of property:

Physical bullying involves force or bodily harm that includes but is not limited to behaviors such as hitting, punching, or kicking another person.

Verbal bullying is oral or written communication by the perpetrator against a student that causes harm such as taunting, name calling, threatening or offensive written notes or hand gestures, and inappropriate sexual comments.

Relational behaviors are designed by a perpetrator to harm the reputation and relationships of a student. Direct relational bullying includes efforts to isolate the targeted youth by preventing interactions with their peers. Indirect relational bullying is comprised of spreading false and/or harmful rumors, publicly writing derogatory comments, or posting embarrassing images in a physical or electronic space without the student's permission or knowledge.

Damage to property includes theft, alteration, or damaging of the target youth's property by the perpetrator to cause harm.

Prevalence and Effect

In the USA the most common forms of bullying are "verbal insults, name calling and nick names, hitting, direct aggression, theft, threats, spreading rumors, and social exclusion or isolation" (UNESCO, 2017). Even though cyberbullying is not mentioned as a popular form of bullying, it should definitely be noted. In fact, in a meta-analysis of 80 studies analyzing bullying involvement rates (for both bullying others and being bullied) for 12–18-year-old students, there was a reported mean prevalence rate of 35% for traditional bullying involvement and 15% for cyberbullying involvement (Modecki, Minchin, Harbaugh, Guerra, & Runions, 2014). Additionally, approximately 80 percent of all high school students have encountered being bullied in some form online (Bullying Statistics, n.d.). Sanchez and Cerezo (2010) examined the prevalence of primary school children's involvement in bullying. They found that for younger students who bullied and were bullied there tended to be a higher incident among those with special needs and immigrants.

There are several underlying causes or risk factors for becoming a victim to bullying. The most vulnerable student populations with the highest risk for bullying are those who have indicators such as low socioeconomic status; ethnic, linguistic, or cultural differences; migration or displacement; and poverty (UNESCO, 2017). A survey of 100,000 bullied youth revealed that 25% were bullied because of physical appearance, 25% because of gender and sexual orientation, 25% because of ethnicity or natural origin, and 25% for other reasons (UNICEF, 2014). According to the CDC, boys are more likely to experience physical bullying from another student, while girls are more likely to experience verbal and relational bullying (Centers for Disease Control and Prevention, 2016). Also, girls are at a higher risk of cyberbullying associated with sexual abuse than boys (UNICEF, 2014). In relation to race and ethnicity, ethnic minorities are more likely to become victims of bullying (Dake, Price, & Telljohann, 2003). Further, youth with disabilities are bullied more than their peers (Carter & Spencer, 2006).

The effects on bullying are profound. The most devastating effect is suicide. The term, "bullycide, is a hybrid of bullying and suicide to explain when someone takes their life as a result of being bullied" (Bullying Statistics, n.d.). Unfortunately, children are also at risk for mental health problems such as depression. Likewise, students report loneliness, anxiety, and low self-esteem. Bullying is also associated with behavioral misconduct in the form of "physical fighting, weapon carrying, theft, property damage, substance abuse, cheating, and breaking the law" (Dake, Price, & Telljohann, 2003).

Cost of Bullying

Bullying is more than a social nuisance with unintended emotional cost to its victims. It also has demonstrated long-lasting financial costs to both the individual and institution. While it is difficult to assess the exact cost associated with negative student behaviors, there are obvious indicators of financial losses to schools that include suspensions, expulsions, truancy, dropout, and vandalism (Phillips, 2011). Thus, institutionally, bullying promulgates absenteeism which in turn effects federal funding that schools receive based on average daily attendance. Therefore, lower student attendance results in lower reimbursement rates that can be in the range of hundreds of thousands to millions of dollars annually (Kemp-Graham & Hendricks, 2015). For example, Baams et al. (2017) found that students who were bullied often felt unsafe which led to absenteeism that cost California school districts $276 million. This magnitude of deficits can decrease districts' ability to leverage school budgets for staff and instructional resources necessary for supporting optimal learning environments.

Additionally, being the victim of bullying, the bully, or both significantly impacts overall life outcomes compared to those who are not bullied (Hill, 2013). For the individual, regardless of the role in the bullying behavior, bullying puts adults at risk of negative effects on health, financial, behavioral, and social outcomes (Wolke, Copeland, Angold, & Costello, 2013). The most notable costs are for mental health services for the victim that often span from childhood to adulthood. Bullying causes mental health problems such as depression and anxiety with increased incidents of self-harm and suicide (Wolke, 2014). Further, according to Wolke et al. (2013), the bully-victims, those who have been bullied and inflict bullying, incur the most devastating financial outcomes with them being 19.9% more likely to live in poverty, 22.5% more likely to drop out of high school, 27% more likely not to have a college degree, and 17.9% more likely to get fired from a job. Academic performance is also compromised. Given that victims are more likely to be absent, children are at a greater risk of low standardized test scores and difficulty transitioning to postsecondary institutions.

Cyberbullying also has a fiscal consequence. The unique nature of this type of bullying can have both individual and institutional implications. Schools hold the burden of providing access to social media and Internet outlets where students may practice bullying behaviors. On the other hand, students are held accountable for the offensive behaviors that cause harm to other students. Both are liable for cyberbullying and are subject to the consequences accordingly. As a result, there are legal costs of cyberbullying. These costs have warranted insurance policies specific to impending legal fees, psychological counseling, and public relations damage control (Teensafe, 2017).

Prevention

As we consider the cost of bullying, it would be fitting to discuss the cost benefit of bullying prevention. Since the nature of bullying is multifaceted, the prevention strategies must also be unique, varied, and comprehensive specific to the needs of the school environment. The cost benefit of effective bullying prevention programs has policy and applied practice implications. As such, the scarcity of state, local, and federal resources allocated to school districts justify understanding why prevention works. Evidence significant to this case is the reduction of expulsions, suspensions, and absenteeism compared to the overall cost of implementation dependent on the number of students, teachers, and staff. The cost benefit analysis is important in that it encompasses the program outcomes and impacts along with the cost to implement at the school level (Windber Research Institute, 2016). The Windber

Institute (2016) examined the cost benefit of a 3-year bullying prevention program with a target population of 1.1 million students across three areas: healthcare, schools, and society. The researchers found a cost benefit on a $25.8 million dollar investment as $2.3 million for healthcare and $6.7 million for schools and projected the cost benefit to society as $1.4 million per individual over a lifetime. This study supports the value of mitigating the effects of bullying for students, schools, and the community at large. While this represents one study, it indicates that prevention should be considered as a viable option for decreasing bullying and its effects.

The purpose of bullying prevention is threefold: positively modify school climates to prevent bullying, reduce aggressive behaviors, and promote collective problem-solving that includes students and adults. In order to reduce bullying, schools must determine the extent to which bullying is a problem by measuring student perceptions of bullying behaviors. Further, schools should address school climates by developing interventions aimed at student attitudes that support bullying and encourage school staff to assist students in understanding that it is acceptable to ask for help (Bandyopadhyay, Cornell, & Konold, 2009). Prevention programs that rely solely on education for teachers and students are difficult to implement and prove to be only slightly effective (Ttotfi & Farrington, 2011). Accordingly, the most successful programs are those that are comprehensive including all stakeholders. One of the unfortunate characteristics of school bullying statistics is that in about "85 percent of bullying cases, no intervention or effort is made by a teacher or administration member of the school to stop the bullying from taking place" (Bullying Statistics, n.d.). Without doubt, the prevention of school bullying should be a priority in fostering healthy school environments. However, before schools embark on a school-wide bullying prevention program, there should be a needs assessment to determine the target population, appropriate strategies, implementation plan, and resources available to complete the initiative. For example, the school's assumption could be that the prevalence of bullying occurs with students between 12 and 18 years of age, so a blanket program is created to encompass these ages. However, the results of a formal needs assessment reveal that the school should really begin its efforts with 14 year olds. This is important as it provides a target group within the school and allows the school to leverage necessary resources.

Given that bullying is a public health threat, prevention strategies should be considered a priority for policy reform and designated resources. Bryn (2011) states that prevention efforts must go beyond the preview of school districts toward engagement with the federal government to garner necessary leadership and create a global understanding of next steps. Nationally, all 50 states have developed policies and/or guidelines to address bullying which are disseminated to local school districts (Ansary, Elias, Greene, & Green, 2015). Cornell and Bradshaw (2015) argue that a comprehensive approach that goes beyond the typical bullying prevention strategies that is inclusive of improving student interactions and the school climate is necessary.

Types of Intervention

A unique characteristic of bullying is that regardless of the helplessness and distress students may feel, they often do not tell anyone of the victimization. This poses a particularly difficult challenge for adults and schools that hope to develop and implement comprehensive school-based interventions to decrease the prevalence of bullying. Fonagy et al. (2009) purport that schools must adopt a multicomponent whole school approach that includes anti-bullying activities representative of the entire stakeholder group: students, teachers, and parents. The overall success of school-based programs is contingent on factors such as parent participation and teacher and peer involvement. Additionally, variations of program focus to include considerations for students' behaviors, emotions, and cognitive processes, as well as developmentally appropriate learning environments and curriculum are important (Hallam, 2009).

Several bullying prevention models can be found in the literature. These models often include one or a combination of several program elements: institutionalizing school rules and behavior management processes, integrating a whole school or ecological bullying prevention program, and supervising students and soliciting cooperation among different professionals and between school staff (Centers for Disease Control and Prevention, 2016).

School Rules and Behavior Management

Most schools adopt for stand-alone prevention programs that emphasize change on the individual student based on the implementation of school rules about behavior and how to handle misbehavior (University of California, 2011). The crux of a conducive school climate in supporting the diverse needs of students is the inherent safety within the learning environments and the strength of relationships between students and school staff. An important element in achieving this is to establish school rules that encourage respect, address conflict, and promote desired student behaviors. Bullying is decreased when schools clearly define "norms, goals, values, interpersonal relationships, teaching and learning practices, and organizational structures" (Wang, Berry, & Swearer, 2013, p. 297). School rules provide a common language to identify and deal with bullying behaviors. Rules also set the standard for overall student behaviors at school.

It is necessary for schools and its staff to have systems in place to assist students in mastering behavior management skills toward optimizing their social and emotional development (Waters & Mashburn, 2017). Waters and Mashburn (2017) argue that when students have the capacity to support others who have been bullied and teachers promote the significance of the student's role, the frequency and the intensity of bullying behaviors diminishes. Accordingly, some schools have embedded anti-bullying programs which focus on behavior management into the curriculum. Positive Behavior Intervention Supports (PBIS) is a systemic approach for improving the school climate and facilitating behavior change in the context of a framework that supports a bullying prevention process. Given that this approach is both comprehensive and proactive, it fosters the redevelopment of the entire school environment (Pugh & Chitiyo, 2012). PBIS is also an evidence-based model comprised of key characteristics of an effective bullying prevention program to include principles to teach appropriate behavior, processes to monitor and acknowledge appropriate behavior, instructions to prevent bullying, corrections and consequences for problem behaviors, evaluations of student behavior, and development of a multidisciplinary teams within the school environment (University of California, 2011). Bradshaw et al. (2015) suggest that PBIS demonstrates the possibility of significant results in relation to school climate, bullying, and academic achievement and should be tracked using data systems throughout the implementation process. Data collection during a PBIS process is instrumental in identifying target areas of focus to include both desired and inappropriate student behaviors toward achieving program outcomes (Bradshaw, 2013). The PBIS is implemented across three tiers: school, classroom, and individual. The PBIS multitiered approach complements other models and through careful alignment can be integrated to develop effective bullying prevention programs (Bradshaw, 2013).

Another framework used in schools is social and emotional learning (SEL). SEL enhances the overall school climate by promoting the development of social and emotional skills of students and school staff. Like PBIS, SEL can be embedded into the school's existing framework and/or bullying prevention model. The primary categories of social skills emphasized in the SEL model are self-awareness, self-management, social awareness, relationship skills, and responsible decision-making (University of California, 2011). SEL provides schools with a mechanism to improve students' social and emotional competencies while impacting bullying on individual and peer levels. Thus, SEL has a direct influence on improving student conflict management and problem-solving skills, reducing inappropriate behaviors, and improving academic achievement (Smith & Low, 2013). Smith and Low (2013) recommend that SEL be considered as a component for bullying prevention as oppose to a stand-alone process as most effective programs use a whole school approach. Given that the skills often taught in SEL programs are empathy, emotion management, and social problem-solving toward social competence, students increase their ability to build strong peer relationships (Smith & Low, 2013). Peer relationships are at the root of bullying, specifically to develop friendships and gauge those students who are liked or disliked. Therefore, self-awareness, social awareness, problem-solving, and relationship management prove beneficial in the reduction of bullying in school environments (Espelage, Rose, & Polanain, 2015).

Whole School and Ecological Approach

The whole school and ecological approach deals with understanding the environmental influences that perpetuate violent or aggressive behaviors that are characteristic in instances of bullying among students. In regard to the whole school approach, the focus is on the primary school environment with some consideration to family dynamics. A whole school approach is common strategy whereby the school program is multifaceted, unique to the schools characteristics, and focused on the community-wide change (Olweus, 1994). Often the strategies employed toward increased awareness of bullying are within the existing infrastructure of the school to include but not limited to supervising recess, conducting parent-teacher conferences, establishing classroom rules, and convening classroom meetings (Dake, Price, & Telljohann, 2003). This approach deals with bullying at all stakeholder levels: administrators, teachers, school staff, and students. The most familiar of these programs is the Olweus Bully Prevention Programs. This program emphasizes "not bullying others, including those who are being excluded, helping those being bullied, and telling an adult at school and home if there has been a bullying incident" (Waters & Mashburn, 2017, p. 6).

The next approach is based on Bronfenbrenner's (1979) ecological model where a child is a product of the norms, values, and rules within a system of environments. Thus, a child's behaviors are not only inherent but also influenced by the ecological context of interactions within each environment. Notably, this is the most effective of all bullying prevention models due to the comprehensive nature of the design (Hornby, 2016). According to Cornell and Bradshaw (2015), the social-ecological approach is a heuristic model that takes into consideration the overarching social influences of the entire stakeholder group in addition to individual interventions that are specific to stopping the demonstrated behaviors of the students. This approach to bullying addresses the systemic environmental influences that shape and sustain student behavior (Bradshaw, 2013). The dynamic and reciprocal environmental influences on bullying behaviors are indicative of the attitudes and beliefs of students, schools, peer groups, communities, and the society at large (Smith & Low, 2013). The discreet variables representative within each of these environments contribute to student's bullying behavior and potential responses to the bullying behaviors of others. Therefore, school bullying prevention programs are developed in the context of changing demographics of communities that includes factors such as race, disability, and sexual orientation (University of California, 2011). In order for schools to have the most success with implementing an ecological approach, it requires careful planning to adjust for the nuances within each level and a plan which is flexible enough to adjust for barriers (Hornby, 2016). Lee (2011) argues that each level of the ecological system is critical to prevalence of bullying.

Supervision and School Staff

Schools are expected to supervise students in their care. Even so, most bullying happens out of sight of school staff and administration. There is a high probability for violent or aggressive behaviors to occur when students have freedom to access areas within the school environment without risk of detection from adults. Therefore, part of the staff training required for bullying prevention programs should include formal, written supervision plans with adults assigned to specific areas of the school (Trump, 2011).

School staff are integral to bullying interventions. The typical players in this model are administrators, counselors, and teachers. Teachers have a unique opportunity to work directly with students who are bullied. Even though many students fail to report bullying, teachers often remain the first observers of inappropriate peer-to-peer social behaviors. Therefore, teachers seem to be ideal candidates for implementing successful bullying interventions. However, for some teachers, this may not be the case as research suggests that teachers are actually ineffective change agents in negative or aggressive classroom situations (Veenstra, Lindenberg, Huitsing, Sainio, & Salmivalli, 2014). This is in part because teachers are not always physically present when incidents occur due to proximity and location that include limited supervision of places like playgrounds, hallways, and lunchrooms. It is important to note that teachers recognize the significance of their roles in relation to bullying. However, many grapple with what actually constitutes bullying to include a common and shared operational definition (Craig, Bell, & Leschied, 2011). Thus, teacher interventions are inconsistent in the field with some taking a proactive stance and fostering positive prosocial environments, while others take more reactive approaches. In fact, when teachers are aware of potential bullying, they seldom intervene. Other barriers to staff-focused intervention models are that teacher perceptions of what constitutes bullying differs and/or varies from that of students and some teachers believe that bullying is a normative developmental process. Despite these challenges, schools still opt primarily for this model and earmark bullying prevention resources toward teacher training.

There are studies that clearly identify the value of staff-based interventions. Without doubt, there is a need for heightened awareness, increased classroom supervision, and targeted opportunities for bullying prevention and intervention from school staff. According to Veenstra et al. (2014), incidents of bullying were lowest in classes in which the teacher appeared efficient at combatting bullying. Thus, when school staff foster a positive school climate, students feel protected and supported. Teacher responses to bullying impact student behaviors and overall classroom management. However, teachers need more than knowledge of bullying to be effective in their role, they also require guidelines on how to respond appropriately (Yoon & Bauman, 2014). Yoon and Bauman (2014) argue that the bullying prevention training that teachers receive mainly focuses on general information about bullying with little to no regard to strategies for how to respond or deal with situations in the school setting. Thus, training alone may not be a comprehensive intervention strategy as it is contingent on both the existing attitudes and beliefs of education professionals as well as their understanding of how to prevent bullying in the school environment (Craig, Bell, & Leschied, 2011). This can significantly impact the effectiveness of anti-bullying initiatives. Teachers must attempt to become actively involved in bullying prevention programs. This may involve collaborating with students to create student-centered approaches that improve the school climate (Al-Raqqad, Al-Bourini, Al Talahin, & Aranki, 2017). Demonstrated responsive social support of school staff fosters a positive school environment and encourages bullied students to seek assistance when dealing with negative prosocial situations (Boulton, et al., 2013). Teachers serve as role models for dealing with conflict, accepting individual differences, setting the standard for respectful behaviors, and enforcing the school rules and the consequences for bullying (Wang, Berry, & Swearer, 2013). As such, teachers' positive relationships with students and clear attitudes against inappropriate behavior are key to successful school environments.

Evaluation

The CDC (2016) states that school-based bullying prevention programs are widely implemented but infrequently evaluated. Even though there are several anti-bullying prevention models, the question remains whether these interventions are effective in eliminating bullying and its adverse effects to school climates. In short, how do we know that these programs work and which elements constitute sustainable best practice? While each model addresses varying elements of the overall problem, it is difficult to determine the definitive impact due to inconsistent evaluation practices and variations in methodological quality. In fact, Cornell and Bradshaw (2015) state that the limitations to evaluating anti-bullying programs include narrowed attention on the internal consistency of bullying measures without consideration to reliability overtime and across individuals, demonstrated validity across varied student populations and environments, and the biased effect on measuring bullying programs. This makes it particularly challenging for researchers, policy makers, and practitioners to identify specific evidence-based best practices in the field of bullying prevention (Bradshaw, 2013). Therefore, there is a need for evidence-based examples of optimal bullying prevention and intervention models (UNESCO, 2017). Specific examples of viable anti-bullying models should fully address the unique factors that constitute the prevalence of violent behaviors in schools (Wang, Berry, & Swearer, 2013).

To ameliorate bullying, it is necessary to identify best practices in prevention and intervention specific to characteristics of the various kinds of bullying across the target population of those being bullied. Some programs demonstrate the strength of evaluation offering a glimpse of the benefits in doing so. McElearney et al. (2013) conducted a longitudinal study on the effectiveness of a bullying intervention program that promoted improved peer relationships for students who have been bullied. The findings indicated that school counseling for students was effective in addressing bullying. Thus, the systematic evaluation proved evidence-based for adult-led interventions that support bullying as well as the benefits of whole school approaches (McElearney, Adamson, & Bunting, 2013). Hallam (2009) evaluated the Social and Emotional Aspects of Learning (SEAL) program that focused on the social, emotional, and behavioral skills of primary children. The pre- and post-questionnaires illustrated that 90% of teachers noted student improvement overall. In another study, a bullying prevention program using a video discussion model was evaluated finding that students increased their knowledge about bullying, victimization, and seeking help (Migliaccio & Raskauskas, 2013). Further, Menard and Grotpeter (2014) conducted an evaluation across 5 years of Bully-Proofing Your School (BPYS), a school-based intervention program designed to reduce bullying. The evaluation proved that BPYS was effective in reducing bullying behaviors, promoting student's understanding of the bullying at school, and increasing student perceptions of school safety. Overall, the characteristics of each of these studies do not lead to the road map for what makes an effective bullying prevention program. However, they do demonstrate the value of an integrated evaluation process for prevention and intervention models in relation to identifying effective programmatic elements. This is also illustrated in Vreeman and Carroll's (2007) review of 26 effective bullying prevention programs across five types of interventions: curriculum, whole school, social skill groups, mentoring, and social work support. Interestingly, less than half of these programs involved controlled evaluations with bullying as an outcome. However, while many evaluations may not be evidence that school-wide interventions eliminate bullying, they do provide evidence of how the interventions impact the student's thoughts and feelings about bullying (Vreeman & Carroll, 2007). The identification of these key components and strategies are integral to bullying prevention research as well as the catalyst for an evidence-based framework.

Despite these findings, the overall evaluation reviews of bullying prevention and intervention programs have mixed findings as none prove to totally eliminate bullying. In fact, most studies do not measure whether bullying is eliminated in the school but instead focuses on such variables as the number of teachers trained, implementation of school rules, and whether a defined program is in place. In addition, other relevant factors include program elements and implementation as well as the role of the school climate on the impact of the bullying prevention program (Low & Van Ryzin, 2014). Such emphases influence the scope of assessment that lead to sufficient program evaluation. Likewise, many programs use bullying assessment tools such as self-report rating scales, student interviews, and student observations to identify and measure effective school-based strategies and techniques that lack rigorous evaluation (Blake, Banks, Patience, & Lund, 2015). Currently, the most popular assessment of the frequency, type of bullying, and how students respond to bullying is the Olweus Bully/Victim Questionnaire (Bandyopadhyay, Cornell, & Konold, 2009). This assessment focuses on how well the intervention increased awareness of bullying problems in students and adults within schools and encouraged adult involvement in resolving the problems. However, this survey fails to establish validity because it relies solely on the accuracy of students' self-reporting of bullying (Lee & Cornell, 2010). This example demonstrates the need for researchers to continue to evaluate the overall effectiveness of programs in the context of such instruments as they are often the first tools of assessment when developing school-wide prevention strategies.

According to Ansary et al. (2015) successful bullying prevention programs have a program philosophy, long-term commitment to effective program implementation, assessment and sustainability, and clear and consistent strategies of what to do when bullying occurs. Yet, these programs demonstrate small margins of success in the reduction of bullying behaviors from school settings. Perhaps this is due to ineffective comprehensive evaluation strategies that are designed to measure eliminating bullying from school environments resulting from the prescribed interventions. Even though there is consistency with programs meeting the desired outcomes, there are significant variations in bullying programs in relation to the type, components used, time commitment, and which stakeholders are involved directly and indirectly (Menard & Grotpeter, 2014). There is also the question of generalization of appropriate socio-emotional competency across environments, specifically the home. Bradshaw (2015) argues that while bullying prevention program outcomes can be achieved, variations in the implementation and compliance to the prevention model influence behavioral outcomes in real-world applications. Unfortunately, current evaluations of bullying prevention programs do not demonstrate sustainability of prosocial behaviors across the students' primary environments (home, school, and community). Ttotfi and Farrington (2011) reviewed bullying prevention approaches and affirmed the benefits of evaluation in understanding the efficacy of bullying prevention programs in schools. The review involved 53 programs of which 44 evaluations showed that school-based bullying prevention programs were effective. Even though contemporary research identifies key program elements that improve student behavior to include behavior management, school rules, teacher training and parent support, comprehensive evaluation of bullying prevention initiatives is needed to test and isolate the critical components of effective bullying prevention programs (Ttotfi & Farrington, 2011).

Conclusion

Bullying is a systemic problem within schools that causes long-lasting effects on students' physically, socially, and emotionally. Certainly, most would agree that students should be privy to and benefit from schools which foster safe learning environments conducive to promoting student's overall physical and mental health. The imminent cost of bullying has led to school-based interventions and anti-bullying policies nationwide. So, how do schools ameliorate the prevalence of bullying? Bullying prevention programs provide students with coping strategies for varied social situations as well as mechanisms that promote social competence in relation to building and sustaining healthy relationships with their peers and adults. Many schools have certainly attempted to remedy the devastating outcomes of bullying through concerted efforts that include strategies and policies specific to prevention and intervention. The problem is that while there are such activities in most school, it is not clear of whether these models actually work. Thus, given the number of school-based bullying prevention programs, it is difficult to discern which is most effective in improving school climate and more importantly eliminating bullying and other violent behaviors perpetuated by students (Bradshaw, 2015). Therefore, researchers should strive to not only support the development of strategies and techniques specific to eliminating bullying but also inform the body of knowledge in the field of bullying prevention by clearly identifying what works through comprehensive evaluation.

References

Al-Raqqad, H., Al-Bourini, E., Al Talahin, F., & Aranki, R. (2017). The impact of school bullying on students' academic achievement from teachers point of view. *International Education Studies, 10*(6), 44–50.

Ansary, N., Elias, M., Greene, M., & Green, S. (2015). *Best practices to address (or reduce) bullying in schools*. Thousand Oaks: Sage Publications, Inc.

Baams, L., Talmage, C., & Russell, S. (2017). Economic costs of bias-based bullying. *School Psychology Quarterly, 32*(3), 422–433.

Bandyopadhyay, S., Cornell, D., & Konold, T. (2009). Validity of three school climate sales to access bullying, agressive attitudes, and help seeking. *School Psychology Review, 38*(3), 338–355.

Blake, J., Banks, C., Patience, B., & Lund, E. (2015). School-based mental health professionals bullying assessment practices: A call for evidence-based bullying assessment guidelines. *Professional School Counseling, 18*(1), 136–147.

Boulton, M., Murphy, D., Lloyd, J., Besling, S., Coote, J., Lewis, J., … Walsh, L. (2013, April). Helping counts: Predicting children's intentions to disclose being bullied to teachers from prior socila support experiences. *British Educational Research Journal, 39*(2), 209–221.

Bradshaw, C. (2013). Preventing bullying through positive behavioral interventions and supports (PBIS): A multitiered approach to prevention and integration. *Theory Into Practice, 52*, 288–295.

Bradshaw, C. (2015). Translating research to practice in bullying prevention. *American Psychologist, 70*(4), 322–332.

Bradshaw, C., Pas, E., Debnam, K., & Johnson, S. (2015). A focus on implementation of positive behavioral interventions and supports in high schools: association with bullying and other indicators of school disorder. *School Psychology Review, 44*(4), 480–498.

Bronfenbrenner, U. (1979). *The ecology of human development: Experiments by nature and design*. Cambridge, MA: Harvard University Press.

Bryn, S. (2011). Stop bullying now! A federal campaign for bullying prevention and intervention. *Journal of School Violence, 10*, 213–219.

Bullying Statistics. (n.d.). *Bullying and suicide*. Retrieved 30 July 2017, from Bullying Statistics: Antibullying help, facts, and more: www.bullyingstatistics.org

Carter, B., & Spencer, V. (2006). The fear factor: Bullying and students with disabilities. *International Journal of Special Education, 21*(1), 11–23.

Centers for Disease Control and Prevention. (2016). *Youth Risk Behaviro Surveillance*. Atlanta: CDC.

Centers for Disease Control and Prevention, C. (2016). *Understanding Bullying: Fact Sheet*. Atlanta: The Centers for Disease Control.

Cornell, D., & Bradshaw, C. (2015). From a culture of bullying to a climate of support: The evolution of bullying prevention and research. *School Psychology Review, 44*(4), 499–503.

Craig, K., Bell, D., & Leschied, A. (2011). Pre-service teachers knowledge and attitudes regarding school-based bullying. *Canadian Journal of Education, 34*(2), 21–33.

Dake, J. A., Price, J. H., & Telljohann. (2003, May). The nature and extent of bullying at school. *Journal of School Health, 73*(5), 173–180.

Espelage, D., Rose, C., & Polanain, J. (2015). Social-emotional learning program to reduce bullying, fighting, and victimiztion among middle school students with disabilities. *Remedial and Special Education, 36*(5), 299–311.

Fonagy, H., Twemlow, S., Vernberg, E., Nelson, J., Dill, E., Little, T., & Sargent, J. (2009). A cluster randomised control trial of child focused psychiatric consultation and a school systems-focused intervention to reduce agression. *Journal of Child Psychology and Psychiatry, 50*(5), 607–616.

Gladden, R., Vivolo-Kantor, A., Hamburger, M., & Lumpkin, C. (2014). *Bullying surveillence among youths:Unifor definitions for public health and recommended data elements*. Atlanta: National Center for Injury Prevention and Control, Centers for Disease Control, United States Department of Education.

Hallam, S. (2009, June). An evaluation of the social and emotional aspects of learning (SEAL) programme: Promoting positive behaviro and well-being in primary school children. *Oxford Reviee of Education, 35*(3), 313–330.

Hill, C. (2013, October 16). *Personal finance: Economic cost of childhood bullying*. Retrieved 29 Oct 2017, from Market Watch: http://www.marketwatch.com/story/bullied-children-grow-up-to-be-poorer-adults-2013-10-15

Hornby, G. (2016). Bullying: An ecological approach to intervention in schools. *Preventing School Failure, 60*(3), 222–230.

Kemp-Graham, K., & Hendricks, L. (2015). The socio-emotional and finacial cost of bullying. *Journal of Bullying and Social Aggression, 1*(1), 1–3.

Lee, C. (2011). An ecological systems approach to bullying behaviors among middle school students in the United States. *Journal of Interpersonal Violence, 26*(8), 1664–1693.

Lee, T., & Cornell, D. (2010). Concurrent validity of the Olweus Bully/Victim Questionnaire. *Journal of School Violence, 9*, 56–73.

Low, S., & Van Ryzin, M. (2014). The moderating effect of school climate on bullying prevention efforts. *School Psychology Quarterly, 29*(3), 306–319.

McElearney, A., Adamson, G. S., & Bunting, B. (2013, January). Impact evaluation of a school-based counseling intervention in northern Ireland: Is it for pupils who have been bullied? *Child Care Practice, 19*(1), 4–22.

Menard, S., & Grotpeter, J. (2014). Evaluation of bully-proofing your school as an elementary school antibullying intervention. *Journal of School Violence, 13*, 188–209.

Migliaccio, T., & Raskauskas, J. (2013, April). Small-scale bullying prevention discussion video for classroom: a preliminary evaluation. *Children and Schools, 35*(2), 71–81.

Modecki, K., Minchin, J., Harbaugh, A., Guerra, N., & Runions, K. (2014, June 6). Bullying prevalence across context: A Meta-analysis measuring cyber and traditional bullying. *Journal of Adolescent Health, 55*, 602–611.

Olweus, D. (1994). Annotation: Bullying at shool: Basic facts and effects of a school based intervention program. *Journal of Child Psychology and Psychiatry, 35*(7), 1171–1190.

Phillips, R. (2011, February 2). School violence: The finacila cost of bullying, violence, and vandalism. *Slate*. Retrieved from Community Matters: http://www.community-matters.org

Pugh, R., & Chitiyo, M. (2012). The problem of bullying in school and the promise of positive behaviour supports. *J Res Spec Educ Needs, 12*(2), 47–53.

Sanchez, C., & Cerezo, F. (2010). Personal and social characterstics of schoolchildren involved in bullying in promary education. *Educational Psychology, 8*(3), 1015–1032.

Smith, B., & Low, S. (2013). The role of social-emotional learning in bullying prevention efforts. *Theory Into Practice, 52*, 280–287.

Teensafe. (2017). Retrieved 29 Oct 2017, from Teensafe: Protecting your most valuable treasure: http:www.teensafe.com

Trump, K. (2011, November/December). Create an antibullying program with resources you have. 35–38.

Ttotfi, M., & Farrington, D. (2011). Effectiveness of school-based programs to reduce bullying: a systematic and meta-analysic review. *Journal of Experimental Criminology, 7*, 27–56.

U.S. Department of Education. (2016). *Student reports of bullying: Results from the 2015 school crime supplemant ti the national crime victimization survey*. Washington, DC: U.S Department of Education.

UNESCO, UN. (2017). *School violence and bullying: Global status report*. Paris: United Nations Educational Scientific and Cultural Organization.

UNICEF. (2014). *Hidden in plain sight: A statistical analysis of violence against children*. New York: UNICEF.

University of California. (2011). *Embedding bullying interventions into a comprehensive system of student and learnign supports*. Center for Mental Health in Schools. California: University of California.

Veenstra, R., Lindenberg, S., Huitsing, G., Sainio, M., & Salmivalli, C. (2014). The role of teachers in bullying: The relation between antibullying attitudes, efficacy, and efforts to reduce bullying. *Journal of Educational Psychology, 106*(4), 1135–1143.

Vreeman, R., & Carroll, A. (2007, January). A systemic reveiw of school-based interventions to prevent bullying. *Arch Pediatric Adolescence Medicine, 161*, 78–88.

Wang, C., Berry, B., & Swearer, S. (2013). The critical role of school climate in effective bullying prevention. *Theory Into Practice, 52*, 296–302.

Waters, S., & Mashburn, N. (2017). An investigation of middle school teachers' perceptions on bullying. *Journal of Social Studies Education Research, 8*(1), 1–34.

Windber Research Institute. (2016). *The cost benefit of bullying prevention: A first time analysis of savings*. Center for Health Promotion and Disease Prevention. Highmark Foundation.

Wolke, D. (2014, April). *The long-term cost of bullying*. Swindon: Economic and Social Research Council.

Wolke, D., Copeland, W., Angold, A., & Costello, J. (2013). Impact of bullying in childhood on adult health, wealth, crime, and social outcomes. *Psychology Science, 24*(10), 1958–1970.

Yoon, J., & Bauman, S. (2014). Teachers: A critical but overlooked component of bullying prevention and intervention. *Theory Into Practice, 53*, 308–314.

Chapter 2
Predictors of Bullying Behavior: An Adlerian Approach

Susan E. Henderson, Reade Dowda, and Rebecca A. Robles-Piña

From an Adlerian theoretical perspective, a loving family would foster social interest, and their children would be less likely to engage in "socially useless" behaviors, such as bullying, drinking alcohol, and smoking. Adler's theory about inferiority complex and the use of bullying to attain a better identity is questioned because it seems that students who feel very good about their relationship with parents as well as students who feel that their parents control too much of their lives are just as likely to bully. Similarly, Adler's theory about social interest is debatable since students who feel good about themselves and their good social standing in school as well as those who perceive favorable opinions from their teachers are likely to bully. Recommendations for counseling students about bullying are discussed.

The purpose of this chapter is to (a) examine the existing systemic literature on the effects that family, school, individual, and substance abuse factors have on bullying, (b) define bullying, (c) define the gap in the literature, and (d) use Adler's theory of individual psychology as a theoretical framework for explaining the empirical results. Further, the purpose is to use a large database for providing empirical evidence to determine which of the predictors explain most of the variance on bullying. Finally, recommendations for adding to best counseling practices in bullying from an Adlerian perspective will be noted.

Bullying is such a significant concern in the United States that since 2007, 35 states have enacted anti-bullying laws to address the problem of bullying in public schools (Srabstein, Berkman, & Pyntikova, 2008). There are other considerations to address, for example, Jordan and Austin (2012) asserted that when bullying stems from a difference in gender, ethnicity, race, sexual orientation, disability, or nationality, then bullying becomes a civil rights issue. Bullying can affect all students, for

S. E. Henderson · R. A. Robles-Piña (✉)
Department of Counselor Education, Sam Houston State University, Huntsville, TX, USA
e-mail: EDU_RAR@shsu.edu

R. Dowda
Clinical Mental Counseling Program, Fort Hays State University, Hays, KS, USA

J. U. Gordon (ed.), *Bullying Prevention and Intervention at School*,
https://doi.org/10.1007/978-3-319-95414-1_2

example, students who are victims of bullying are not the only ones who suffer negative effects. Leung and To (2009) indicated that students who perceived frustration and fear without the support of their peers utilized bullying as a way to release the emotions caused by the strain they endured from interpersonal stress, family stress, and academic stress. Ultimately, Flaspohler, Elfstrom, Vanderzee, Sink, and Birchmeier (2009) reported that there is a correlation between developing negative consequences later in life and being both a victim and a perpetrator of bullying; therefore, bullying is a problem that needs to be addressed to help perpetrators as well as victims.

Bullying is a serious systemic problem (Casebeer, 2012), and multiple factors contribute to the problem, including schools (Allison, Roeger, Smith, & Isherwood, 2014; Felix & McMahon, 2007; Robles-Piña, Nichter, & Campbell-Bishop, 2004; Robles-Piña & Denham, 2012; Twemlow & Sacco, 2013), individuals (Coloroso, 2011; Joaquim, 2014), families (Allison et al., 2014), peers (Felix & McMahon, 2007), and social media (Twemlow & Sacco, 2013). According to systems researchers (Seifert, Schmidt, & Ray, 2012), violent behavior is not caused by any one factor but includes factors that interact with one another and may prevent individuals from full participation in society. Additionally, Casebeer (2012) described bullying as a systemic problem that "requires a deep understanding of the multiple variables with which it is associated" (p. 165), thus, the importance of studying bullying from a systemic perspective.

Because bullying is not just an individual problem, there are a host of negative outcomes. For example, school shootings, suicide, and academic difficulties have been found to impact all students who are involved in bullying (Casebeer, 2012). Similarly, students who display bullying behaviors are more likely to have conflicted family relationships (Low & Espelage, 2013; Mohapatra et al., 2010), substance abuse issues (Litwiller & Brausch, 2013; Radliff, Wheaton, Robinson, & Morris, 2012), lower levels of life satisfaction (Allison et al., 2014), and display negative attitudes toward themselves (Leung & To, 2009). Further, easy access to social media increases the likelihood that bullying is inescapable and can affect students continuously (Burton, Florell, & Wygant, 2013).

Gaps in the Literature

Children often use social aggression to fit in at school and gain attention or status. It is important to recognize what contributes to bullying behaviors if we are to create a peaceful environment at school. To effectively implement prevention measures, we must gain a better understanding of the complex nature of bullying and how bullying is affected by multiple factors. There is an extensive body of literature about bullying in relation to correlates and predictors (Allison et al., 2014; Leung & To, 2009; Litwiller & Brausch, 2013; Low & Espelage, 2013; Mohapatra et al., 2010; Radliff et al., 2012), but there is limited research regarding multiple environmental factors associated with bullying. Because adolescents influence and are influenced by different environments, it is important to obtain a holistic approach in understanding bullying. Furthermore, for prevention programs to be effective, the complexities involved in bullying in multiple environments must be considered (Swearer & Hymel, 2015). Our study adds to the extant literature in that it investigates the relationship between bullying behavior and substance abuse and family, individual, and school factors. Additionally, there is a dearth of literature concerning Adlerian psychology (Watts, 2013a) as a means of explaining bullying behavior. Our article addresses all these issues to add to the existing body of literature.

Bullying

In this study, bullying encompasses all types of bullying including physical, emotional, and cyberbullying. Olweus and Limber (2010) defined bullying as "intentional, repeated, negative behavior" (p. 125) perpetrated by a person of more power to a person of lesser power. Physical bullying includes being hit, kicked, or pushed. Emotional bullying is verbal abuse such as being made fun of or called names. Emotional bullying includes indirect bullying, social aggression, and relational aggression. Indirect bullying causes psychological harm by intentionally ignoring or excluding students (Srabstein, et al., 2008). Social aggression is manipulative and may include gossiping, spreading rumors, or social exclusion. This type of non-physical bullying can devastate students by disrupting relationships or damaging social status (Archer & Coyne, 2005; Froeschle & Riney, 2008). Relational aggression is the intent to harm another person through the manipulation of a relationship (Low, Polanin, & Espelage, 2013). While physical aggression is normally dyadic, relational aggression often involves spreading rumors or excluding students from a group (Low et al., 2013).

Cyberbullying

Cyberbullying allows bullying behavior to continue outside of school. Electronic communication is used in cyberbullying, and students use text messages, social media, and other forms of communication to engage in cyberbullying (Hinduja & Patchin, 2013; Low & Espelage, 2013), which can be dangerous because they can be saved, forwarded, and taken out of context (Allen, 2012). Burton et al. (2013) remarked that students who engaged in cyberbullying were more likely to engage in traditional bullying. Although the definition of bullying varies, the common theme in bullying behavior is that students with more physical or social power use this to negatively impact a student who is physically weaker or less popular.

Literature Review

The literature explored for this study was on how the following factors and theory impacted bullying: (a) family, (b) school, (c) personal, (d) substance abuse, and (e) Adlerian psychology.

Family Factors

Understanding the impact of relationships is essential for recognizing, understanding, preventing, and responding to bullying (Low & Espelage, 2013). The following researchers discussed family factors that affected bullying. For example, Bibou-Nakou, Tsiantis, Assimopoulos, and Chatzilambou (2013) conducted a qualitative study in which 90 students were involved in 14 focus groups, and they documented that students with less supportive parental relationships were more likely to engage in bullying behavior. Other researchers support this finding in their meta-analysis of 8985 children and adolescents where they found a weak but positive correlation of $r = 0.17$ between parenting style and bullying (Kuppens, Laurent, Heyvaert, & Onghena, 2013). Goswami (2012) utilized a sample of 4673 secondary students and found a small, but significant, association between family relationships and bullying with a correlation coefficient of $r = -0.013$. Family relationships, being bullied by peers, and unfair treatment by adults can all have a negative impact on the mental health of children (Goswami, 2012; Leung & To, 2009). Murray-Harvey and Slee (2010) conducted a study with 888 middle school students and noted that teacher, peer, and family relationships all had direct effects on psychological health, social and emotional adjustment ($R^2 = 0.64$), and bullying. Low and Espelage (2013) sampled 1023 middle school students and indicated that maladaptive social interaction in the home predicted a wide array of aggression in school. They further outlined that males engaged in more verbal and relational aggression, while females manifested higher levels of cyberbullying. Seeds, Harkness, and Quilty (2010) found that abuse perpetrated by fathers and peers was more directly related to a child's sense of not belonging and feeling disconnected from their world. Further, they indicated that these children were more likely to receive a diagnosis of depression because they perceived their fathers and peers to be unavailable. Stevens, de Bourdeauhuij, and van Oost (2002) conducted a study where they surveyed 1719 fifth- and sixth-grade students and 1401 parents. They asked children and parents to self-identify whether they were bullies, bullied, or not involved in bullying and compared the groups' responses on various factors related to family life. They found a significant difference ($p < 0.0001$) between children in the areas of (a) family cohesion, (b) family expressiveness, (c) family conflict, and (d) personal family relationships. Stevens et al. (2002) indicated that the results they found were consistent with previous studies conducted; however, they made a distinction that there were not many studies at the time examining the perceptions of the parents of bullies. When they analyzed the differences between parental groups, they found very little difference in reports about family life but some significant differences ($p < 0.05$) in avoidance of relationships between parents and children. Thus, predominantly, the literature on family and bullying indicates that family dynamics affect bullying; however, whether it has a negative or positive impact remains unclear.

School Factors

Bullying is often used as a tool by adolescents to combat feelings of inferiority. Adolescents engage in socially useless behaviors, a term coined by Adler (Adler & Fleischer, 1988a), such as social aggression to damage the reputation of peers. Students in school might try to achieve a higher social rank by making others look more negative (Froeschle & Riney, 2008). Strong, positive, and supportive relationships between teachers and students are beneficial to reduce bullying and to foster safer schools (Elsaesser, Gorman-Smith, & Henry, 2013; Murray-Harvey & Slee, 2010; Robles-Piña et al., 2004; Robles-Piña & Denham, 2012). Similarly, children who view their friendships more negatively are more likely to be dissatisfied with school (Goswami, 2012). Thus, peer relationships within the school significantly impact bullying. In fact, researchers (Froeschle & Riney, 2008) found that people who engage in bullying behavior may actually have difficulty in forming peer relationships in the future. Researchers de Bruyn, Cillessen, and Wissink (2010) commented that of the 1207, 13–14-year-old adolescents in their study, females bullied less than males ($\beta = -0.29$). Peer acceptance (students in class accept me as I am) significantly negatively predicted bullying behavior ($\beta = -0.47$), whereas perceived popularity significantly positively predicted bullying behavior ($\beta = 0.60$). One of the least studied factors is that of bullying behavior being related to the amount of pressure from schoolwork. Bibou-Nakou et al. (2013) reported that respondents in their qualitative study claimed that pressure from teachers and the school system to work hard and compete with other students caused stress that led to bullying behavior.

Personal Factors

Family relationships, being bullied by peers, and unfair treatment by adults can all have a negative impact on the mental health of children (Goswami, 2012). Students ($N = 4331$) who engaged in bullying behavior reported lower life satisfaction ($M = -0.11$, SE = 0.02) than students who did not bully ($M = 0.08$, SE = 0.01), $F(1, 4310) = 70.20$, $p < 0.001$, partial $n^2 = 0.02$. Furthermore, victims of bullying reported less life satisfaction ($M = -0.15$, SE = 0.02) than non-victims ($M = 0.12$, SE = 0.02), $F(1, 4310) = 138.31$, $p < 0.001$, partial $\eta^2 = 0.03$. Students who were victims, but not perpetrators, reported more perceived social support from teachers than did students who bullied. Overall, being a victim or engaging in bullying contributed to lower life satisfaction and a reduced perception of social support. However, reporting more peer support brought the correlation between being victimized and life satisfaction from $r = -0.27$ to $r = -0.19$ (Flaspohler et al., 2009). Thus, supportive peer relationships alleviate the negative impacts of bullying.

Substance Abuse Factors

People need to belong to a group to survive. Behaviors that contribute to the group are socially useful, while behaviors that do not contribute to the group are socially useless (Carlson, Watts, & Maniacci, 2006). A thorough search of the literature resulted in a limited number of studies addressing substance abuse and bullying. However, of the studies found that examined the influence of substance use on bullying behaviors, a strong relationship existed between substance use and bullying (Luukkonen, Riala, Hakko, & Räsänen, 2010; Radliff et al., 2012; Smalley, Warren, & Barefoot, 2017).

In one study (Radliff et al., 2012) researchers studied 74,247 middle and high school students on the relationship between bullying behavior and substance abuse (cigarettes, alcohol, and marijuana). They indicated that both bullies and the victims of bullying reported higher substance abuse than students who reported not being involved in bullying behavior, with bullies reporting the highest use. These researchers further elucidated the relationship between bullying behavior and substance abuse with Cramer's V values of 0.19 and 0.16 for middle school respondents and 0.14 and 0.17 for high school respondents. All students reported higher alcohol than cigarette use. In a second study, Luukkonen et al. (2010) examined 508 adolescents at an inpatient psychiatric hospital and noted that substance-related disorders were significantly higher ($p < 0.001$) among adolescents who reported bullying others (59.5%) than those who reported being victims (23.0%). Boys who reportedly bullied had higher percentages of daily smoking (85.7% vs. 59%) and weekly alcohol use (57% vs. 23%) than boys who claimed to be victims. Girls who reportedly bullied also had higher percentages of daily smoking (96.7% vs. 58.3%) and weekly alcohol use (60% vs. 34.8%) than girls who claimed to be victims. Finally, Durand et al. (2013) provided a review of relevant research regarding substance use and bullying. Durand and colleagues concluded that bullying is associated with substance use on some level; however, the direction of the association is unclear (2013).

Theoretical Framework of the Study

Individual psychology, also referred to as Adlerian psychology (Carlson et al., 2006), was used as the theoretical framework for this research because many aspects of individual psychology, such as social interest and lifestyle, assist in explaining bullying behavior. For example, Adler believed that human behavior is motivated by social interest that begins during a child's formative years, and he and Fleischer (1988b) wrote that children justify their own desires for power based on the behaviors of their role models.

> Right from the start, the human psyche has a tendency to strive toward the goal of total superiority. When from the behavior of adults, as in our time, the child senses the increased bellicosity, the tyranny, the will to power, he will perceive this behavior as justification for his own desire for power, especially if he even experiences this pressure in his upbringing. (p. 420)

We argue that this desire for power might translate into utilizing bullying behavior as a way to gain social status and manipulate one's identity in school. Social interest is related to the development of identity. "A personality construct related to both social interest and common sense is how one's identity is defined" (Forman & Crandall, 1991, p. 142). These authors further affirmed that a person's social identity is manifested in roles and relationships. Adler and Fleischer (1988a) stated, "A human being does not exist for himself alone. He is not apart from others" (p. 407). The social identity of our target population of children and adolescents in grades six through ten is the students' identity at school. Social identity at school is founded in relationships and is associated with the relationships formed while attending school. Essentially, peer relationships at school are important in developing and maintaining positive psychological health (Elsaesser et al., 2013; Murray-Harvey & Slee, 2010; Ojanen, Smith-Schrandt, & Gesten, 2013).

Lifestyle, also known as a person's cognitive life map, includes subjective, self-created goals. If a person feels inferior, common to most human beings, this can lead to faulty thinking about oneself and others and can eventually lead to self-defeating behaviors (Mosak & Maniacci, 2011). Furthermore, the need to belong directly impacts mental well-being. People who experience a need to belong are better adjusted than those who do not feel a need to belong (Ferguson, 2010). Both home and school environments are perfect examples of where children must balance the need to belong, to find an identity, and to feel superior to their peers. Dilmac (2009) reported that students who bully are attempting to satisfy their need for superiority by engaging in aggressive and manipulative behaviors. Children who are dissatisfied with life, family relationships, or school might become discouraged and view their social environments as hostile (Adler, 2011; Adler & Fleischer, 1988a). Having a negative view of one's environment could lead to socially useless behaviors, such as bullying. We believe that children who engage in bullying behaviors feel inferior to their peers and seek superiority by displaying aggressive behavior.

Study Purpose

The purpose of our study was to examine bullying from an Adlerian perspective and to include systemic factors (i.e., family, school, substance use, and individual) that are included in the microsystem and mesosystem (Espelage, Hong, Rao, & Thornberg, 2015) that impact bullying behaviors. We sought to determine which risk and protective factors predicted bullying behavior in the past last 30 days for students in grades six through ten. The identification of specific systemic risk and protective factors helps with the development of intervention programs in the school and community to protect children against bullying. Family therapists, school personnel, and intervention program developers can target problem areas once they know the systems that influence bullying behaviors.

Research Question

Which of the following predictors (a) life satisfaction, (b) satisfaction with family relationships, (c) parent/guardian is loving, (d) parent/guardian understands my problems, (e) parent/guardian tries to control the things I do, (f) parent/guardian treats me like a baby, (g) teacher's opinion of school performance, (h) present feelings about school, (i) students in class accept me as I am, (j) amount of pressure from schoolwork, (k) how often smoked cigarettes in the past 30 days, and (l) how often drunk alcohol in the past 30 days are most influential in predicting bullying behavior in middle and high school students?

Method

Prior to the initiation of the study, we were granted permission by the university Institutional Review Board (IRB) for collection of data. Because we used a large dataset and did not collect data, no consent forms were needed. Quantitative data, collected from the 2005–2006 Health Behaviour in School-aged Children (HBSC; Iannotti, 2012) study, were used to determine predictors of bullying behavior.

Dataset

The HBSC study, conducted every 4 years, is based on independent national surveys of students ages 11–15 in more than 40 participating countries. The data in the current study is from the 2005–2006 study conducted in the United States and was funded by the US Department of Health and Human Services, National Institutes of Health, Eunice Kennedy Shriver National Institute of Child Health and Human Development, and the US Department of Health and Human Services Health Resources and Services Administration, Maternal and Child Health Bureau.

Since 1982, the HBSC cross-national study has been sponsored by the World Health Organization (WHO) Regional Office in order to identify and monitor attitudes and behaviors of youth who pose psychological and behavioral health risks during early adolescence. The purpose of sampling this age group is because early adolescence marks a time when there are more physical, emotional, social, and intellectual challenges. It is during this time that individuals struggle with their identity, peer group, and gaining independence from their family (Iannotti, 2012).

Sampling

In order to obtain a nationally representative sample, sampling was conducted over three stages: districts, schools, and classes. The "Primary Sampling Units (PSUs) were stratified within each Census Division" (Iannotti, 2012, p. 2). One or more public school districts were in each PSU. The list of schools was obtained from Quality Education Data, Inc. (QED) and was divided by urban and rural. Grouping occurred where each PSU had at least ten schools. A sample of 100 PSUs was selected from the 1540 PSUs that were created. In order to ensure similar probability of selecting a private, Catholic, or public school, similar sampling was conducted with private and Catholic schools. The second sampling stage consisted of sampling by district. The final count of schools participating in the study was 227, with the majority of districts having between 1 and 3 schools in the final sample. The last sampling stage consisted of sampling classes in each school, with all students completing the survey in the sampled class. Both the age-based (11, 13, and 15 years) and grade-based (6–10) samples were used "to provide precision estimates of ±3 percent at 95 percent confidence for student characteristics" of either groups (Iannotti, 2012, p. 2). In order to obtain a representative sample, African-American and Hispanic students were oversampled. Approximately 75% of the sampled schools had two classes selected, and approximately 17% percent had one class that was included in the final sample. The total sample consisted of 227 schools with 9227 participating students in grades six through ten.

Participants

The target population was students in grades 6 through 10 in public, Catholic, and other private schools in the 50 states as well as the District of Columbia. Thus, the 9227 participants in the study were a representative sample from all public, private, and Catholic schools in the 50 states and District of Columbia. However, we included only the participants who had complete data. Therefore, in order to maintain integrity of the data, participants with missing data on the variables of interest were removed, decreasing the sample size to 8277. Additionally, the total sample was further reduced because we wanted to analyze only those participants who admitted to bullying another student in the past 2 months. Once these participants were removed from the analysis, the final sample size was 2946. The demographic characteristics of the final sample are shown in Table 2.1.

Table 2.1 Participants' demographic characteristics in analysis

Characteristic		*n*	%
Gender			
	Males	1532	52.00
	Females	1410	47.90
	Missing	4	0.10
Ethnicity			
	Hispanic	725	24.50
	Not Hispanic or Latino	2155	73.20
	Missing	68	2.30
Race			
	White	1312	44.50
	Black or African-American	563	19.10
	Asian	78	2.60
	American Indian or Alaskan native	55	1.90
	Native Hawaiian or other Pacific islander	22	0.70
	Other	605	20.50
	Two or more races	292	9.90
	Missing	19	0.60
Grade level			
	6th grade	635	21.60
	7th grade	618	21.00
	8th grade	665	22.60
	9th grade	503	17.10
	10th grade	525	17.80
Total			
	Participants in analysis	2946	100.0

Note: The sample size includes removed cases from the analysis for the variables of interest because of incomplete data

The responses for race and ethnicity were weighted and combined into five categories (White, Black, or African-American, Hispanic, Asian, and Native American). The weighted totals corresponded to the National Center for Education Statistics web site. Thus, the weights adjust the totals for race/grade to correspond to national totals.

Instrumentation

The HBSC (Iannotti, 2012) self-report questionnaire asked questions about multiple factors related to emotional and physical development, relationships with family and friends, and school-related issues. The questionnaire took approximately 45 min to complete and contained over 80 questions. Students answered the questions in a regular classroom setting while school personnel (e.g., teacher, nurse, counselor) administered the survey. The procedures for the questionnaire were scripted and were read to the students. There were two separate versions of the questionnaire for sixth-grade students, one for seventh-, eighth-, and ninth-grade students and one for tenth-grade students. Thus, there were four versions of the questionnaire.

Variables

The 12 independent or predictor variables (IVs) and the dependent variable (DV) for our study, along with how the data were collected and mean and standard deviations, are as follows. There were two statements that used continuous data (i.e., life satisfaction and satisfaction with family relationships), and scores with lower numbers indicated negative responses (e.g., worst possible life, very bad relationships), while higher scores indicated positive responses (e.g., best possible life, very good relationships). Three statements related to family factors used a three-point Likert-type scale (i.e., parent/guardian is loving, parent/guardian understands my problems, parent/guardian tries to control things I do, and parent/guardian treats me like a baby), and lower numbers indicated higher agreement (i.e., 1 = almost always). Three statements related to school factors used a four-point Likert-type scale (e.g., teacher's opinion of your school performance, present feelings about school, amount of pressure from schoolwork), and lower numbers indicated higher agreement (i.e., 1 = almost always). One school-related question was a five-point Likert-type scale question (e.g., students in my class accept me as I am), and the substance use statements were measured on a seven-point Likert-type scale (i.e., past 30 days how often smoked cigarettes, past 30 days how often drunk alcohol), and higher numbers indicated more agreement. The dependent variable, how often have you bullied another student in the last 30 days, was defined by a five-point Likert-type scale. Participants who answered "1 = I haven't bullied another student" were excluded from the analysis; lower numbers indicated less amounts of bullying.

Reliability

The 2005–2006 Health Behaviour in School-Aged Children survey provided stable and consistent results for several reasons. First, sampling was conducted in three stages: districts, school, and classes. Additionally, participants in the study were representative from all public, private, and Catholic schools in the 50 states and District of Columbia. Weights were applied to correspond to the National Center for Education Statistics web site. Thus, the weights adjusted the totals for race/grade to correspond to national totals. The procedures for administration also were standardized in that the instructions were scripted and read to the students prior to the administration of the questionnaire. Regarding the data collection, the Inter-university Consortium for Political and Social Research (ICPSR), part of the Institute for Social Research at the University of Michigan, performed consistency checks on data collection, standardized missing values, and checked for undocumented or out-of-range codes (Iannotti, 2012). Roberts et al. (2009) stated that in order for the survey to be translated for use in over 40 countries, the questions were translated, then translated back into English, and compared against the original survey. The back translations were then checked again by researchers and translators.

Validity

The self-report questionnaire states that it was designed to measure multiple factors related to emotional and physical development, relationships with family and friends, and school-related issues. Additionally, these questions were piloted at national and international levels (Roberts et al., 2009). Lastly, the instrument is well known and robust and has been in use since 1982. Thus, because the HBSC is reliable and valid, it is a psychometrically sound instrument.

Data Analysis

We used standard multiple regression with 12 IVs relating to individual factors (e.g., life satisfaction, past 30 days how often smoke cigarettes, past 30 days how often drunk alcohol), family factors (e.g., satisfaction with family relationships, parent/guardian is loving, parent/guardian understands my problems, parent/guardian tries to control the things I do, parent/guardian treats me like a baby), and school factors (e.g., teacher's opinion of your school performance, present feelings about school, students in class accept me as I am, amount of pressure from schoolwork) in order to determine which variables were stronger predictors of bullying behavior (e.g., how often have you bullied another student in the last 30 days). Multiple regression was chosen for the analysis because it can be used to predict multiple values on a dependent variable and it provides a least square solution that predicts values of a DV from IVs. Additionally, multiple regression reduces errors in predicting response variables (Mertler & Vannatta, 2013).

Results

Preliminary Data Analysis

We used SPSS version 21 (IBM, 2012) for data analysis. Because we were only interested in participants with complete data, those participants with incomplete or missing data were manually removed from the database in order to maintain integrity of the data. Additionally, responses of non-bullying behavior were removed from the analysis. This resulted in a final sample of 2946 for analysis. The data were examined for the following assumptions: (a) multivariate outliers, (b) linearity, (c) normally distributed data, and (d) homoscedasticity. According to the Mahalanobis distance, there were no multivariate outliers, and the scatterplot indicated linear data. Conversion of skewness and kurtosis coefficients to *z* scores indicated that the majority of the variables were not normally distributed as they were not within the limits of +3 and − 3 (Tabachnick and Fidell, 2007). However, the analysis continued due to the explanation from the central limit theorem that states that as sample size increases the distribution of means will increasingly approximate a normal distribution around the true population mean ($n = 2946$). Additionally, moderate violations of normality assumptions may be ignored many times with large sample sizes (Lumley, Diehr, Emerson, & Chen, 2002; Tabachnick & Fidell, 2007). The last assumption of homoscedasticity was met because the scatterplot indicated that residuals were scattered and were not clustered in certain areas (Mertler & Vannatta, 2013). Based on the assumptions that were met and the central limit theorem regarding normality of data, we proceeded with the standard multiple regression analysis.

Secondary Analysis

We conducted a standard multiple regression to determine which IVs previously discussed predicted bullying behavior. Initially, multicollinearity was checked to determine if any variables were explaining the same phenomenon (Mertler & Vannatta, 2013), and there was no evidence. After consulting the model summary, an R^2, the coefficient of determination (0.062), was examined and indicated that a small to medium effect size (Cohen, 1988) of 6% of the variance of bullying was explained by the combination of the predictors. Subsequently, regression results indicated that the overall model significantly predicted bullying behavior ($R^2 = 0.062$, $F[12, 2933] = 16.242, p < 0.001$).

The next step in interpretation was to determine which variables statistically significantly predicted the most variance by examining the β (beta) weights. The β (beta) weights, strength of the relationship between a given predictor and the criterion in standardized form ($M = 0$, $\text{SD} = 1$), were interpreted. The formula produced by the statistically significant predictors was $Z_{\text{Bullying}} = 2.14_{\text{constant}} + (0.125_{\text{drank alcohol}}) + (0.078_{\text{parent is loving}}) + (0.075_{\text{present feelings about school}} + (0.058_{\text{smoked cigarettes}}) + (-0.052_{\text{parent treats me like baby}}) + (0.039_{\text{teacher's opinion of your school performance}})$.

Out of the 12 predictors, 6 were statistically significant at <0.05 (Table 2.2). Of those six predictors, five had positive β weights, indicating that a positive increase in the predictor indicated a positive increase in the DV, bullying behavior. By order of influence of β weights, the following were noted to positively increase bullying: (a) drinking alcohol about one or twice a week ($m = 1.97$, $\text{sd} = 0.03$), (b) parents who almost always display loving behavior ($m = (1.27$, $\text{sd} = 0.52)$, (c) student who likes school a little bit ($m = 2.33$, $\text{sd} = (0.02)$, (d) students who have smoked once or twice ($m = 1.63$, $\text{sd} = (0.03)$, and (e) a good and above average teacher's opinion of

Table 2.2 Significant predictors on bullying another student

Predictor		*B*	SE *B*	*β*	t	*p*	Partial	Part	Tolerance
	(constant)	2.14	0.160		13.404	0.000			
Parent/guardian: is loving		0.140	0.037	0.078	3.755	0.000	0.069	0.067	0.732
Parent/guardian: treats me like a baby		−0.067	0.027	−0.052	−2.520	0.012	−0.046	−0.045	0.759
Teacher's opinion of your school performance		0.040	0.020	0.039	2.009	0.045	0.037	0.036	0.855
Present feelings about school		0.076	0.020	0.075	3.815	0.000	0.070	0.068	0.823
Past 30 days how often: smoked cigarettes		0.035	0.014	0.058	2.548	0.011	0.047	0.046	0.618
Past 30 days how often: drunk alcohol		0.075	0.014	0.125	5.522	0.000	0.101	0.099	0.621

Note: $R^2 = 6\%$

school performance ($m = 2.30$, sd = 0.02). One (1) predictor was inversely related to bullying; those students who indicated that their parents "sometimes treats me like a baby" ($m = 2.42$, sd = 0.01) were most likely to bully.

Discussion

Our study supports and extends previous research in this area. We used a representative sample of 2946 children and adolescents in grades six through ten. It is important to note that all students in our study reported bullying to some degree and the following findings report varying degrees of bullying with the predictors. In summary of our findings, from an individual perspective there were two individual predictors indicating that adolescents who drank alcohol and smoked were more likely to bully. From a family perspective, adolescents who felt good about their relationship with their parents as well as parents who treated them like babies were more likely to bully. Finally, from a school perspective, students who feel they like school a little bit and who receive good opinions from their teachers are likely to bully.

Regarding individual factors, the findings from this study indicated that the largest predictor indicated that students who drink alcohol have the highest likelihood of bullying, and the fourth largest predictor was smoking. These findings were supported by researchers who stated that both perpetrators and victims were more likely to drink alcohol than respondents not involved in bullying behavior (Luukkonen et al., 2010; Radliff et al., 2012). Further, these findings were supported by researchers who found that both perpetrators and victims of bullying behavior were more likely to smoke cigarettes than participants not involved in bullying behavior (Luukkonen et al., 2010; Radliff et al., 2012). Thus, in counseling students about bullying, alcohol and smoking are factors that need to be included in an integrated program. Adler would suggest investigating how drinking alcohol, smoking, and violence were viewed in the family dynamic to increase power.

From a family perspective, our findings fall in between, with some students indicating that when they had good parental support, they bullied and when they felt that their parents were overly involved "treated them like babies," they were also likely to bully. Our findings were somewhat conflicted with existing research since the majority of the research indicates that more supportive parental relationships are correlated with less bullying (Bibou-Nakou et al., 2013; Goswami, 2012; Leung & To, 2009; Low & Espelage, 2013). However, there is some research that is congruent with our findings. For example, Kuppens et al. (2013) found that parental psychological control was weakly but positively correlated to aggression in the schools. Consistent with our findings were those of de Bruyn et al. (2010) who found that popularity in school positively impacted bullying behavior. From an Adlerian perspective, there needs to be a balance in parent-child interactions about acquisition of power, and this finding indicates that more research is needed.

Regarding school factors and bullying, the existing research has indicated that positive relationships with teachers and positive feelings about school decrease bullying behavior (Elsaesser, et al., 2013; Flaspohler et al., 2009; Murray-Harvey & Slee, 2010). Furthermore, decreased feelings of belongingness to school and decreased teacher affiliation was associated with more bullying (Espelage et al., 2015). Our findings partially contradict these findings since students who felt good about school and who perceived favorable opinions from their teachers reported they were likely to bully. Adler's theory would likely explain this finding by indicating that social identity and power acquisition within the school system are due to a delicate balance. Due to the contradictory nature of these findings, more research is needed to replicate these findings.

While this study's findings supported some of the existing literature about bullying, there were some unique findings. First, in contrast to other studies, this one used 12 variables to find out which ones were most predictive. Evident was the fact that counseling intervention programs should include many factors as no one single factor predicts bullying behavior. Second, most predictors had received support from other studies; however, the predictor that has not been researched as much is the one about students who feel that their parents baby them too much are more likely to bully. Third, our findings were in contradiction to some of the existing research, and further research is needed to replicate these findings. What is evident, however, is that multiple factors are involved in explaining bullying. In sum, our original hypothesis that students who bully are seeking superiority was not borne out because some students who felt good about their relationships with teachers and parents also admitted to bullying. Thus, there is a need to examine power superiority and social status further.

It is recommended that counseling programs include improving social relationships between child and parent, increasing discussions about power and bullying, and emphasizing allowing children to learn from their mistakes as well as their successes. The three most important predictors that should be addressed when counseling about bullying should be (a) use of alcohol, (b) improving relationships with parents, and (c) improving students' relationship with school and teachers. It is recommended that counseling programs include a drug prevention program including family and school issues as part of a comprehensive program that follows the four phases of Adlerian counseling. Further, the findings of this study indicate that both negative and positive factors affecting relationships between students, teachers, and parents must be examined.

Adlerian Counseling Recommendations

In the reorientation phase, the counselor assists the student to form attainable goals, such as "I know that I made a mistake by hitting Jimmy, but I have learned that I can talk to Jimmy and tell him that I do not like it when he makes fun of me and I plan to do this in the future."

The following phases of Adlerian counseling of (a) relationship, (b) analysis/assessment, (c) insight/interpretation, and (d) reorientation/reeducation (Watts, 2013a) will be used for making recommendations for counseling students about bullying. Establishing a relationship with the client is the most important aspect of counseling (Thomas, 2006) and one that is focused on encouragement (Carlson et al., 2006). It becomes essential for counselors to examine students' cognitions, thoughts, and values and encourage students to change how they view power attainment. Through assessment of early childhood recollections about first memories, the counselor seeks to understand where the student learned about seeking power and identity formation. Subsequently, through encouragement the student can be taught to seek an identity that does not include violence or bullying. In the insight phase, the counselor forms hypotheses based on the information gathered from student and uses a question format that seeks validation of the hypothesis from the client. For example, the counselor could state "Could it be that…" or "Is it possible that you learned that the only way to be heard is to yell?" as interpretation. This will help the student understand where the values and beliefs have come from and what needs to change. Based on our clinical experience, reflecting "as if" has proven to be a beneficial intervention in that students can describe a past situation and process what they would like to have done differently. Reflecting "as if" expands on the more well-known Adlerian intervention of acting as if in which an Adlerian counselor may ask how the student would like to have behaved differently if he or she was acting as the person he or she wanted to be (Watts, 2013b).

References

Adler, A. (2011). *Understanding human nature: The psychology of personality* (trans: Colin Brett.). Oxford, England: Oneworld Publications. (Original work published 1927).

Adler, A., & Fleisher, L. (1988a). Problem Children. *Individual Psychology: The Journal of Adlerian Theory, Research & Practice, 44*(4), 406–416.

Adler, A., & Fleisher, L. (1988b). The child's inner life and a sense of community. *Individual Psychology: The Journal of Adlerian Theory, Research & Practice, 44*(4), 417–423.
Allen, K. P. (2012). Off the radar and ubiquitous: Text messaging and its relationship to 'drama' and cyberbullying in an affluent, academically rigorous US high school. *Journal of Youth Studies, 15*(1), 99–117. https://doi.org/10.1080/13676261.2011.630994
Allison, S., Roeger, L., Smith, B., & Isherwood, L. (2014). Family histories of school bullying: Implications for parent-child psychotherapy. *Australasian Psychiatry, 22*(2), 149–153. https://doi.org/10.1177/1039856214520791
Archer, J., & Coyne, S. M. (2005). An integrated review of indirect, relational, and social aggression. *Personality and Social Psychology Review, 9*(3), 212–230. https://doi.org/10.1207/s15327957pspr0903_2
Bibou-Nakou, I. I., Tsiantis, J. J., Assimopoulos, H. H., & Chatzilambou, P. P. (2013). Bullying/victimization from a family perspective: A qualitative study of secondary school students' views. *European Journal of Psychology of Education, 28*(1), 53–71. https://doi.org/10.1007/s10212-011-0101-6
Burton, K. A., Florell, D., & Wygant, D. B. (2013). The role of peer attachment and normative beliefs about aggression on traditional bullying and cyberbullying. *Psychology in the Schools, 50*(2), 103–115. https://doi.org/10.1002/pits.21663
Carlson, J., Watts, R. E., & Maniacci, M. (2006). *Adlerian therapy: Therapy and practice*. Washington, DC: American Psychological Association.
Casebeer, C. M. (2012). School bullying: Why quick fixes do not prevent school failure. *Preventing School failure: Alternative Education for Children and Youth, 56*(3), 165–171. https://doi.org/10.1080/1045988X.2011.633283
Coloroso, B. (2011). Bully, bullied, bystander … and beyond. *Education Digest, 77*(4), 36–39.
Cohen, J. (1988). *Statistical power analysis for the behavioral sciences* (2nd ed.). Hillsdale, NJ: Lawrence Erlbaum.
de Bruyn, E. H., Cillessen, A. N., & Wissink, I. B. (2010). Associations of peer acceptance and perceived popularity with bullying and victimization in early adolescence. *The Journal of Early Adolescence, 30*(4), 543–566. https://doi.org/10.1177/0272431609340517
Dilmaç, B. (2009). Psychological needs as a predictor of cyber bullying: A preliminary report on college students. *Kuram Ve Uygulamada Eğitim Bilimleri, 9*(3), 1307–1325.
Durand, V., Hennessey, J., Wells, D. S., Crothers, L. M., Kolbert, J. B., Lipinski, J., & Hughes, T. L. (2013). Bullying and substance use in children and adolescents. *Journal of Addiction Research & Therapy, 4*(4), 1–6. https://doi.org/10.4172/2155-6105.1000158
Elsaesser, C., Gorman-Smith, D., & Henry, D. (2013). The role of the school environment in relational aggression and victimization. *Journal of Youth and Adolescence, 42*(2), 235–249. https://doi.org/10.1007/s10964-012-9839-7
Espelage, D. L., Hong, J. S., Rao, M. A., & Thornberg, R. (2015). Understanding ecological factors associated with bullying across the elementary to middle school transition in the United States. *Violence and Victims, 30*, 470–487. https://doi.org/10.1891/0886-6708.VV-D-14-00046
Felix, E. D., & McMahon, S. D. (2007). The role of gender in peer victimization among youth: A study of incidence, interrelations, and social cognitive correlates. *Journal of School Violence, 6*(3), 27–44.
Ferguson, E. D. (2010). Adler's innovative contributions regarding the need to belong. *Journal of Individual Psychology, 66*(1), 1–7.
Flaspohler, P. D., Elfstrom, J. L., Vanderzee, K. L., Sink, H. E., & Birchmeier, Z. (2009). Stand by me: The effects of peer and teacher support in mitigating the impact of bullying on quality of life. *Psychology in the Schools, 46*(7), 636–649. https://doi.org/10.1002/pits.20404
Forman, B. D., & Crandall, J. E. (1991). Social interest, irrational beliefs, and identity. *Individual Psychology: Journal of Adlerian Theory, Research & Practice, 47*(1), 141–149.
Froeschle, J. G., & Riney, M. (2008). Using Adlerian art therapy to prevent social aggression among middle school students. *The Journal of Individual Psychology, 64*(4), 416–431.
Goswami, H. (2012). Social relationships and children's subjective well-being. *Social Indicators Research, 107*(3), 575–588. https://doi.org/10.1007/s11205-011-9864-z

Hinduja, S., & Patchin, J. W. (2013). Social influences on cyberbullying behaviors among middle and high school students. *Journal of Youth and Adolescence, 42*(5), 711–722. https://doi.org/10.1007/s10964-012-9902-4

Iannotti, Ronald J. (2012) Health Behavior in School-Aged Children (HBSC), 2005–2006. ICPSR28241-v1. Ann Arbor, MI: Inter-university Consortium for Political and Social Research [distributor]. doi:https://doi.org/10.3886/ICPSR28241.v1. Accessed 29 Feb 2012.

IBM Corp. (2012). *IBM® SPSS® Statistics for Windows, (Version 21.0) [Computer software].* Armonk, NY: IBM Corp.

Joaquim, C. (2014). Developmental stage of performance in reasoning about school bullying. *Behavioral Development Bulletin, 19*(2), 81–99.

Jordan, K., & Austin, J. (2012). A review of the literature on bullying in U.S. schools and how a parent–educator partnership can be an effective way to handle bullying. *Journal of Aggression, Maltreatment & Trauma, 21*(4), 440–458. https://doi.org/10.1080/10926771.2012.675420

Kuppens, S., Laurent, L., Heyvaert, M., & Onghena, P. (2013). Associations between parental psychological control and relational aggression in children and adolescents: A multilevel and sequential meta-analysis. *Developmental Psychology, 49*(9), 1697–1712. https://doi.org/10.1037/a0030740

Leung, C., & To, H. (2009). The relationship between stress and bullying among secondary school students. *New Horizons in Education, 57*(1), 33–42.

Litwiller, B., & Brausch, A. (2013). Cyber bullying and physical bullying in adolescent suicide: The role of violent behavior and substance use. *Journal of Youth & Adolescence, 42*(5), 675–684. https://doi.org/10.1007/s10964-013-9925-5

Low, S., & Espelage, D. (2013). Differentiating cyber bullying perpetration from non-physical bullying: Commonalities across race, individual, and family predictors. *Psychology of Violence, 3*(1), 39–52. https://doi.org/10.1037/a0030308

Low, S., Polanin, J. R., & Espelage, D. L. (2013). The role of social networks in physical and relational aggression among young adolescents. *Journal of Youth and Adolescence, 42*(7), 1078–1089. https://doi.org/10.1007/s10964-013-9933-5

Lumley, T., Diehr, P., Emerson, S., & Chen, L. (2002). The importance of the normality assumption in large public health data sets. *Annual Review Public Health, 23*, 151–169.

Luukkonen, A. H., Riala, K. K., Hakko, H. H., & Räsänen, P. P. (2010). Bullying behaviour and substance abuse among underage psychiatric inpatient adolescents. *European Psychiatry, 25*(7), 382–389. https://doi.org/10.1016/j.eurpsy.2009.12.002

Mertler, C. A., & Vannatta, R. A. (2013). *Advanced and multivariate statistical methods* (5th ed.). Glendale, CA: Pyrzcak Publishing.

Mohapatra, S., Irving, H., Paglia-Boak, A., Wekerle, C., Adlaf, E., & Rehm, J. (2010). History of family involvement with Child Protective Services as a risk factor for bullying in Ontario schools. *Child & Adolescent Mental Health, 15*(3), 157–163. https://doi.org/10.1111/j.1475-3588.2009.00552.x

Mosak, H. H., & Maniacci, M. (2011). Adlerian psychotherapy. In R. J. Corsini & D. Wedding (Eds.), *Current psychotherapies* (9th ed., pp. 67–112). Belmont, CA: Brooks/Cole.

Murray-Harvey, R., & Slee, P. T. (2010). School and home relationships and their impact on school bullying. *School Psychology International, 31*(3), 271–295. https://doi.org/10.1177/0143034310366206

Ojanen, T., Smith-Schrandt, H. L., & Gesten, E. (2013). Associations among children's social goals, responses to peer conflict, and teacher-reported behavioral and academic adjustment at school. *Journal of Experimental Education, 81*(1), 68–83. https://doi.org/10.1080/00220973.2011.635167

Olweus, D., & Limber, S. P. (2010). Bullying in school: Evaluation and dissemination of the Olweus Bullying Prevention Program. *American Journal of Orthopsychiatry (Wiley-Blackwell), 80*(1), 124–134. https://doi.org/10.1111/j.1939-0025.2010.01015.x

Radliff, K. M., Wheaton, J. E., Robinson, K., & Morris, J. (2012). Illuminating the relationship between bullying and substance use among middle and high school youth. *Addictive Behaviors, 37*(4), 569–572. https://doi.org/10.1016/j.addbeh.2012.01.001

Roberts, C., Freeman, J., Samdal, O., Schnohr, C., Looze, M., Nic Gabhainn, S., ... the HBSC Methods Group Development. (2009). The health behavior in school-aged children (HBSC) study: Methodological developments and current tensions. *International Journal of Public Health, 54*(2), 140–150. https://doi.org/10.1007/s00038-009-5405-9

Robles-Piña, R. A., Nichter, M., & Campbell-Bishop, C. (2004). Assessment of counselors' and teachers' perceptions about bullying in schools. *The Journal of At-Risk Issues, 10*(1), 11–19.

Robles-Pina, R. A., & Denham, M. A. (2012). School resource officers for bullying interventions: A mixed methods analysis. *Journal of School Violence, 11*(1), 38–55. https://doi.org/10.1080/15388220.2011.630311

Seeds, P. M., Harkness, K. L., & Quilty, L. C. (2010). Parental maltreatment, bullying, and adolescent depression: Evidence for the mediating role of perceived social support. *Journal of Clinical Child, & Adolescent Psychology, 29*(5), 681–692.

Seifert, K., Schmidt, R., & Ray, K. (2012). *Youth violence: Theory, prevention, and intervention.* New York: Springer Publishing.

Smalley, K. B., Warren, J. C., & Barefoot, K. N. (2017). Connection between experiences of bullying and risky behaviors in middle and high school students. *School Mental Health, 9*(1), 87–96. https://doi.org/10.1007/s12310-016-9194-z

Srabstein, J. C., Berkman, B. E., & Pyntikova, E. (2008). Antibullying legislation: A public health perspective. *Journal of Adolescent Health, 42*(1), 11–20. https://doi.org/10.1016/j.jadohealth.2007.10.007

Stevens, V., de Bourdeauhuij, I., & van Oost, P. (2002). Relationship of the family involvement to children's involvement in bully/victim problems at school. *Journal of Youth and Adolescence, 31*(6), 419–428.

Swearer, S. M., & Hymel, S. (2015). Understanding the psychology of bullying: Moving towards a social-ecological diathesis-stress model. *American Psychologist, 70*(4), 344–353. https://doi.org/10.1037/a0038929

Tabachnick, B. G., & Fidell, L. S. (2007). *Using multivariate statistics* (5th ed.). Boston, MA: Allyn & Bacon.

Thomas, M. L. (2006). The contributing factors of change in a therapeutic process. *Contemporary Family Therapy, 28*, 201–210.

Twemlow, S. W., & Sacco, F. C. (2013). Bullying is everywhere: Ten universal truths about bullying as a social process in schools & communities. *Psychoanalytic Inquiry, 33*(2), 73–89. https://doi.org/10.1080/07351690.2013.759484

Watts, R. E. (2013a). Adlerian counseling. In B. J. Irby, G. Brown, R. Lara-Alecio, & S. A. Jackson (Eds.), *The handbook of educational theories* (pp. 459–472). Charlotte, NC: Information Age Publishing.

Watts, R. E. (2013b). Reflecting as if. *Counseling Today, 55*(10), 48–53.

Chapter 3
Bibliotherapy as a Strategy for Bullying Prevention

Kristen Pennycuff Trent and Stephanie J. Richards

Bibliotherapy as a Strategy for Bullying Prevention

In the United States, 49 out of 50 states have passed legislation requiring public schools to take action to stop bullying (U.S. Department of Health & Human Services, 2014). While some districts have school-wide anti-bullying campaigns, many do not. Teachers hoping to change bullying behaviors may be limited by increased pressure to focus solely on academic content (Cox & Witko, 2011). As an alternative, the purpose of this study was to examine the impact of teachers' use of high-quality children's books with anti-bullying messages during the existing read-aloud time. This process of bibliotherapy is one strategy for helping students create schema for facing bullies (Esch, 2008; Enteman, Murnen & Hendricks, 2005; Rowan, 2007; Schechtman, 2006). Consider the following vignettes.

Seated in a rocking chair, Ms. Carlie reads from *The Recess Queen* (O'Neill, 2002) "Jean doesn't push kids and smoosh kids…," and her first graders chorally chant "…lollapaloosh kids, hammer 'em, slammer 'em, kitz and kajammer 'em." Ms. Carlie continues "Because she's having too much fun rompity romping with her FRIENDS. Bouncity, kickity, swingity, hoppity, skippety, jumpity, ringity, zingity…," and the students join in for a rousing "YESSSSSSS!!!" Ms. Carlie then asks her students to Think-Pair-Share (Lyman, 1981) what gave Katie Sue the courage to stand up to Mean Jean and then befriend her. Heads together, partners are deep in conversation about the anti-bullying tactics the main character used to engage the antagonist in positive ways.

In a middle school in the same district, Mr. Lopez has his sixth graders arranged in neat rows as they do a quick write after he read-aloud *Mr. Lincoln's Way* (Polacco, 2001). Students refer to individual copies of the text that Mr. Lopez typed the night before as they find textual evidence and write independently. "Two more minutes,"

K. P. Trent · S. J. Richards (✉)
Curriculum and Instruction, Tennessee Tech University, Cookeville, TN, USA
e-mail: srichards@tntech.edu

J. U. Gordon (ed.), *Bullying Prevention and Intervention at School*,
https://doi.org/10.1007/978-3-319-95414-1_3

Mr. Lopez guides, "And then be prepared to share how Mr. Lincoln redirected Eugene's bullying behaviors so he could see how to treat everyone with kindness and respect."

Both teachers are immersing their students in bibliotherapy, which we define as the process of engaging students in reading or listening to exemplary texts carefully curated by an educator to correspond with aspects of socio-emotional development including, but not limited to, bullying. The use of bibliotherapy as a strategy for preventing bullying behaviors is explored in this chapter through theoretical background, examples of model practice in a research study, analysis and discussion of results, and conclusions and recommendations.

Theoretical Background of Bibliotherapy

History of Bibliotherapy The practice of using literature to improve healthy development has long been documented. The entrance to the library of Thebes was inscribed as "the healing place for the soul" (Afolayan, 1992; Reed, 2015; Sullivan and Strang, 2002). Aristotle wrote of the "therapeutic value of reading" (Afolayan, 1992, p. 137), while Shakespeare entreated audiences of "Titus Andronicus" to "Come, and take choice of all my library, and so beguile thy sorrow" (Afolayan, 1992; Dovey, 2015; Johnson, Wan, Templeton, Graham & Sattler, 2001; Sullivan & Strang, 2002). Another inscription in the library of the medieval Abbey of St. Gall in Switzerland reads "the medicine chest for the soul" (Afolayan, 1992; McCulliss, 2012). In 1840, John Galt described the practice of bibliotherapy as a form of treatment for mental illness, but the term was not coined until 1916 when Samuel Crothers wrote of his friend's Bibliopathic Institute in an article entitled "A Literary Clinic" published in *The Atlantic Monthly* (Afolayan, 1992; Beatty, 1962; Dovey, 2015; McCullis, 2012). After World War I, returning soldiers with post-traumatic stress disorder were given books to use as therapy; librarians in the United States received special training on which books to recommend, while Jane Austen was prescribed in the United Kingdom (Dovey, 2015; Reed, 2015).

Bibliotherapy was first documented in grammar school in 1946 when Sister Mary Agnes published a study on the use of literature as a method of overcoming issues with maladjusted children (Johnson, et al., 2001; McCulliss, 2012). The landmark publication, *Bibliotherapy: A Theoretical and Clinical Experimental Study*, by Caroline Shrodes (1950) is considered the first model to outline the process of identification, catharsis, and insight that bibliotherapy can offer (McCulliss, 2012). Later facilitator-led dialogue, guided group discussions, and written exercises were added to the strategy from the fields of psychiatry and counseling (McCulliss, 2012).

Schultheis and Pavlik's *The Classroom Teacher's Manual for Bibliotherapy* (1977) contained ideas for presenting and creating lessons with text as well as assessment methods. Rubin (1979) referred to the goal of bibliotherapy used in school settings as promoting healthy development and potential achievement. Pardeck (1986) advocated for the use of bibliotherapy as a technique to help children navigate needs of development. Ouzts (1991) emphasized the need for students engaging in bibliotherapy to actively participate and interact with supplemental activities instead of solely reading a text. In 1995 Goleman documented the use of bibliotherapy by classroom teachers to decrease bullying behaviors, and Doll and Doll (1997) noted growing use of the strategy by teachers and school personnel in the classroom setting. In the early 2000s several published recommendations for assisting teachers in the evaluation of trade books used for bibliotherapy with bullying prevention (Enteman, Murnen, & Hendricks, 2005; Moulton, Heath, Prater, & Dyches, 2011; Murray, Shea, and Harlin, 2007).

Only in the past 30 years have some experts suggested a dichotomy between *developmental bibliotherapy* used by educators and *clinical bibliotherapy*, practiced by mental health practitioners to reconcile more significant emotional and behavioral complications (Afolayan, 1992; McMillen, 2014). Recently, other categories have emerged. *Reading or suggestive bibliotherapy* is the practice of a well-read individual who suggests texts without engaging the reader in or following up after the process (McMillen, 2014). It can be contrasted with *interactive bibliotherapy* where the reading of the recommended text becomes the focus of discussion and other forms of interaction (McMillen, 2014). With the addition of "self-help books, computer-aided interventions, and virtual reality therapy, the field of bibliotherapy continues to broaden…" (McCulliss, 2012, p. 30).

Recently, bibliotherapy has entered in popular culture as well with the affective reading practice of Ella Berthoud and Susan Elderkin (Dovey, 2015). The two authors of *The Novel Cure: From Abandonment to Zestlessness: 751 Books to Cure What Ails You* (Berthoud & Elderkin, 2014) state that they are "dedicated to fiction as the ultimate cure because it gives readers a transformational experience" (Dovey, 2015, no page). Along with their first book, their latest publication, *The Story Cure: An A-Z of Books to Keep Kids Happy, Healthy and Wise* (Berthoud & Elderkin, 2016a, 2016b), is written in the same genre as a medical reference book with pairings for ailments and suggested texts as remedies (Dovey, 2015). In this latest release, Berthoud and Elderkin (2016a, 2016b) remind us that:

> [b]etween 'Once upon a time' and 'happily ever after' is a land we've all been to. Strange and marvelous things happened there….By the time we come back, brushing the dust off our hats, a new, worldly look in our eye, we alone know what we've seen, experienced, endured. And we've discovered something else, too: that whatever is going on in our actual lives, and whatever we're feeling about it, someone else has felt that way too. We're not alone, after all. (p.1)

Benefits of Bibliotherapy Bibliotherapy is not just something teachers do to make student feel better. It encourages students to safely engage in emotional expression through positive discussion about the characters in a supportive environment (Johnson, Wan, Templeton, Graham, & Sattler, 2001). Research shows that it is an effective strategy in increasing socio-emotional skills and decreasing anxieties (Campbell, 2003; Enteman et al., 2005; Frey, Hirschstein, Snell, Edstrom,

MacKenzie, & Broderick, 2005; Rowan, 2007; Sullivan & Strang, 2002; Thompson, 2009). Forgan (2002) and Frey et al. (2005) used the strategy to help promote problem-solving skills. Others also assert that the practice promotes the development of empathy, an emotion bullies are often lacking (Enteman et al., 2005; Louie, 2005; Murray, Shea, & Harlin, 2006). Goleman (1995) documented fewer cases of physical and verbal bullying in classrooms using bibliotherapy as well as an increase in teachers' abilities to help scaffold conflict resolution among students. Another study found that when students were exposed to a program with bibliotherapy as a key component, there was a decrease in both bullying behaviors and bystanders who were encouraging the acts (Frey et al., 2005). In accordance with the words of Murray, Shea, and Harlin (2006), "We strongly believe that a similar empathetic response to the bully, the bullied, and the bystander can be evoked though the reading, responding, and discussing exemplary, authentic children's literature on bullying" (p. 99).

Curating Exemplary Texts for Bibliotherapy Selecting the right text for the right moment can be intimidating. Berthoud and Elderkin (2014) categorize "overwhelmed by the number of books in the world" as an ailment, and it's easy to see why (p. 286). Those seeking to create a collection of exemplary texts for bibliotherapy should first consider the unique classroom composition, matching characters and plotlines to the needs of individuals and groups (Moulton et al., 2011). One place to begin is to seek annotated bibliographies already crafted from recommended sources such as those listed in the Box 3.1, *Where to Find Exemplary Text for Bibliotherapy*. For example, Bartle's (2016) *Database of Award Winning Children's Literature* has the ability to search over 12,000 books and 142 awards using a variety of search terms including suggested age range or publication year, as well as ethnicity or gender of protagonist. Murray, Shea, and Harlin (2006) remind us that we need a systematic method of evaluation for exemplary text and recommend that teachers ask themselves a series of questions including: "Does this book effectively deal with the issue of bullying? Do the bullying situations portrayed in the book clearly identify the roles of the bully, the bystander, and/or the victim? How accurately does the book represent bullying dynamics?" (p. 99). Others advocate for educators to also examine literature for coping strategies to use when experiencing bullying (Moulton et al., 2011). Teachers may want to spend time immersing themselves in the variety of picture and chapter books so they can carefully categorize exemplary texts for a variety of bullying scenarios. Well-appointed with a curated selection of exemplary texts, Enteman et al. (2005) suggest another question we think is significant: How can this book be used to address bullying in my classroom? As the authors go on to state:

> In the hands of the right teacher at the right moment, a children's book can be a powerful tool for engaging students in dialogue that either ends the bullying or gives victims and bystanders the knowledge and confidence to face it. (Enteman et al., 2005, p. 361)

Implementing Bibliotherapy. In the words of Johnson et al. (2001):

> Bibliotherapy is the process by which teachers, as informed decision makers, select appropriate reading materials and match them to the needs of the individual students to assist them in the development of self-awareness, problem-solving skills, perspective taking, and understanding of problems. (p. 173)

To actively engage students in the bibliotherapy process, teachers should emphasize texts "not as a substitute but as a catalyst for discussion" (Thibault, 2003, no page). Dialogue and interaction are the critical pieces for successful implementation of bibliotherapy, as highlighted in the six guidelines below.

Motivation with Introductory Activities Teachers should select materials, resources, and activities that promote diversity and to which students can relate (Forgan, 2002; Karges-Bone, 2015). Creative dramatics, readers' theater, and puppets can be used to predict what the story will be about and how students can relate it to their own lives. Positive discussion about the characters in a supportive environment is critical for establishing safety for emotional expression by students (Johnson et al., 2001).

Reading Time Bibliotherapeutic text requires longer reading time by at least 25% or more time (Johnson et al., 2001). Teachers should ensure that children have adequate time to read and process the text. Sullivan and Strang (2002) recommend the following questions for maintaining active dialogue during reading:

> What is the story about?
> How does the story make you feel?
> Who is the main character?
> What problem is the main character encountering?
> How did the main character solve the problem?
> If you faced a similar problem, what might you do? (p.80)

Incubation Students should have ample time to develop their thoughts, feelings, and connections to the text. Emotional needs may also require specific encouragement in interactive reading. Positive reinforcement should be used in verbal and nonverbal communication with the student (Johnson et al., 2001).

Follow-Up Discussion Time Being aware of cultural and emotional needs of students, teachers should stimulate discussion with questions that promote higher-level thinking. Student-generated questions should be encouraged and are often perceived as less invasive than teacher-guided questions. At all times, the discussion should be interactive and supportive (Forgan, 2002; Johnson et al., 2001; Sullivan and Strang, 2002).

Evaluation and Closure Students need to evaluate both the process and product of bibliotherapy, as well as self-evaluating their performance. Teachers should model revealing what events occurred in the text, emotions produced by the events, and personal connections to emotions and actions. Authentic follow-up activities should be provided for students to reinforce meaning (Johnson et al., 2001).

Caregiver Involvement Teachers should encourage the home-school connection by sending home copies of the bibliotherapeutic text and offering additional reading selections and meaningful activities caregivers can do at home (Sullivan and Strang, 2002).

As with any teaching strategy or technique, bibliotherapy is not to be entered into lightly. Karges-Bone (2015) cautions teachers to remember sensitivity, confidentiality, and advisability when planning to implement bibliotherapy. Educators should be sensitive to the needs of their students by allowing students to opt out of participation and to be prepared for possibility of an emotional reaction to the content. They should maintain confidentiality by respecting the privacy of both the student and the caregivers. Teachers should also have a thorough knowledge and familiarity with the texts and questions that are being used, as well as considering how the text could be perceived from various cultural lenses (Karges-Bone, 2015).

Model Practice

We have a tradition of curating exemplary texts in our own classrooms for bibliotherapy with students ranging in age from kindergarten to graduate college students. We have long used picture books and novels as a way to engage students in conversation about important topics for discussion. We have found bibliotherapy to be particularly effective for sensitive topics because it allowed students to empathize with characters in conflict and engage in dialogues in a safe environment. Some of the latest statistics show that between 71% and 74% of all students have experienced bullying in their lifetimes and 30 percent of males and 36 percent of females have been cyberbullied in their lifetimes (Pachin & Hinduja, 2016). We devised a study that used bibliotherapy to specifically target bullying in the elementary and middle school setting.

Participants Thirty-four teachers in urban, suburban, and rural areas of two states agreed to participate in a mixed method study. Despite our attempts to extend deadlines and encourage participation, only 20 teachers completed surveys with only 9 sets of matched pairs pre- and post-surveys completed. We believe this may have been because we mailed sets of exemplary text and the Bibliotherapy Reading Guide (BRG) to all who agreed to participate instead of waiting until pre-surveys had been collected. All 20 teachers were included in the qualitative analysis of open-ended responses; however only the subgroup of 9 matched pairs were also analyzed quantitatively. For generalizability, we have chosen to describe each group separately, noting that the subgroup is part of the main population of 20.

Of the 20 teachers whose surveys and anecdotal notes were analyzed qualitatively, 3 taught kindergarten, 3 taught first grade, 5 taught second grade, 1 taught a Comprehensive Disability Class (CDC) for grades 1–3, 3 taught fourth grade, 4 taught sixth grade, and 1 taught eighth grade. They had a range of teaching experience from 1 year to 26 years, with a mean of 3.57 years of experience. One teacher had an associate's degree, while 14 held bachelor's degrees and 5 held master's degrees. Fifteen teachers were from school systems in Tennessee and five were from school systems in Texas. Eight classified their school setting as urban, four as suburban, and eight as rural. Class sizes ranged from 10 students to 103 students, with a mean of 19 and a median of 23.5 students.

Nine teachers completed both pre- and post-surveys for quantitative analysis. Two taught kindergarten, two taught first grade, one taught a Comprehensive Disability Class (CDC) for grades 1–3, three taught fourth grade, and one taught sixth grade. They had a range of teaching experience from 1 year to 25 years, with a mean of 10 years and a mode of 2 years of experience. One teacher had an associate's degree, while five held bachelor's degrees and three held master's degrees. Seven teachers were from school systems in Tennessee and two were from school systems in Texas. Four classified their school setting as urban, two as suburban, and three as rural. Class sizes ranged from 10 students to 103 students, with a mean of 26.8 and a median of 18 students.

Methods Two weeks before implementation, teachers were asked to complete the Bullying Behaviors Survey with Likert-scaled responses and open-ended questions and collect anecdotal data on their perceptions and attitudes toward student bullying behaviors in the classroom, including observed or reported incidences of bullying. Participants then entered into a 10-school-day treatment period in which they read 1 of the 11 provided exemplary texts each day during their scheduled read-aloud time. Selections included ten picture books and one novel. They were encouraged to use any of the texts in any order they deemed appropriate for their particular classroom. During each read-aloud session, participants agreed to use the provided before-, during-, and after-questions included on the Bibliotherapy Reading Guide (BRG) to encourage dialogue and problem-solving about bullying behaviors and related issues. The BRG was designed to include basic comprehension and higher order thinking questions to push the students in their thinking about what actions the bully took, how the bystanders either were or were not involved, how the victim responded to resolve the conflict, and whether adults were consulted to help clear up the conflict. There were also questions that asked the students to think about how they might have handled the situations so that they could look at the story from a personal frame of reference. Teachers were told that use of the Bibliotherapy Reading Guide was the most important aspect of their participation. After the 10-day intervention period, teacher participants wrote anecdotal notes about their observations, perceptions, and any changes in student bullying behaviors in the classroom as well as their own perceptions of self-efficacy. They also completed a second Bullying Behaviors Survey as a posttest.

Instrumentation The Bullying Behaviors Survey was given 2 weeks prior and 2 weeks after implementation. Teachers ranked their perception of frequency and intensity of bullying behaviors of students on a Likert-type scale in categories of name calling, physical violence, social isolation, comments on physical appearance of others, and bystander behaviors. Additionally, participants rated their own familiarity with and confidence in implementation of bullying prevention strategies for general bullying prevention, bibliotherapy, and teaching empathy. Open-ended questions were also answered ranging from current practices related to bullying prevention, bibliotherapy, and empathy building to impact of the intervention on teacher practice and student behavior. Teacher participants also collected anecdotal notes on their perceptions of student behaviors, student behavior changes, and their own self-efficacy both 2 weeks prior to implementing bibliotherapy and 2 weeks after treatment concluded.

Analysis of Results

Data collected from teacher surveys and anecdotal notes were analyzed qualitatively and quantitatively to establish triangulation. Twenty-one pre-surveys and nine post-surveys were completed, and all open-ended questions and anecdotal notes were analyzed using open coding (Corbin & Strauss, 2008). It should be noted that only nine participants completed both pre- and post-surveys despite our multiple attempts to encourage greater response. We attribute this to the fact that the study occurred late in the school year when teachers were overwhelmed with testing and preparations for the end of the term. In fact, one sixth grade teacher noted on her survey "I am not seeing a huge improvement with this. I am inclined to believe this is largely a result of two factors: time and age. Knowing the psychology of this age group, the concern is focused on self and not other. I think by starting this early next year and setting a tone, I could see a difference by the end of the year." Another fourth grade participant wrote "I hope that it [bibliotherapy] has made them stop and think about how their behavior affects others-it is the end of the year so it is hard to make this determination because we are out of our regular routine most days." Because of the limited set of completed survey data, quantitative results of analysis should be very cautiously interpreted.

Quantitative Analysis Eighteen completed pre-surveys and 13 post-surveys were collected despite our attempts to collect more. Only nine matched pairs of pre- and post-surveys were received, and all were analyzed using the Wilcoxon signed-rank test in SPSS for statistical significance. Four concepts were statistically significant: familiarity with bullying prevention methods, confidence in ability to prevent bullying, familiarity with bibliotherapy strategies, and familiarity with strategies to teach empathy. Of the nine sets of completed pre- and post-surveys, seven participating teachers saw an increase in familiarity with methods for preventing bullying, two teachers noted no change, and no teacher reported a decrease in familiarity with prevention methods. A Wilcoxon signed-rank test determined that there was a statistically significant median increase in familiarity methods for preventing bullying (Mdn = 1.000) post-intervention (Mdn = 3.000) compared to pre-intervention (Mdn = 3.000), $z = -2.460$, $p = 0.014$. An additional statistically significant median increase was detected for confidence in ability to prevent bullying (*Mdn* = 1.000) post-intervention (*Mdn* = 4.000) compared to pre-intervention (*Mdn* = 3.000), $z = -1.994$, $p = 0.046$. Six participating teachers saw an increase in confidence with methods for preventing bullying, two teachers noted no change, and one teacher reported a decrease in confidence with bullying prevention methods after intervention. There was also a statistically significant median increase for familiarity with bibliotherapy strategies (*Mdn* = 2.000) post-intervention (*Mdn* = 4.000) compared to pre-intervention (*Mdn* = 1.000), $z = -2.328$, $p = 0.020$. Seven participating teachers saw an increase in familiarity with bibliotherapy strategies, one teacher noted no change, and one teacher reported a decrease in familiarity with bibliotherapy strategies after intervention. Finally, six participating teachers saw an increase in familiarity with strategies to teach empathy, two teachers noted no change, and one teacher reported a decrease in familiarity with strategies to teach empathy. A Wilcoxon signed-rank test determined that there was a statistically significant median increase in familiarity with strategies to teach empathy (*Mdn* = 1.000) post-intervention (*Mdn* = 4.000) compared to pre-intervention (*Mdn* = 3.000), $z = -2.050$, $p = 0.040$. Additional Wilcoxon signed-rank testing revealed no statistically significant median changes in frequency or intensity of student behavior indicators: name calling, social isolation, physical violence, making comments on physical appearance of others, and bystander behaviors. There were also no statistically significant median changes detected for indicators of teacher confidence in applying bibliotherapy strategies and teaching empathy (Table 3.1).

Table 3.1 Pre-post significance levels using Wilcoxon *Z*-scores ($n = 9$)

Variable name	*Z*-score	Significance (two tailed)
Frequency name calling	0.378	0.705
Intensity name calling	0.647	0.518
Frequency social isolation	−1.127	0.260
Intensity social isolation	0.000	1.000
Frequency physical violence	0.000	1.000
Intensity physical violence	−0.828	0.408
Frequency comments on looks	0.322	0.748
Intensity comments on looks	0.408	0.683
Frequency bystander	0.000	1.000
Intensity bystander	0.333	0.739
Familiarity bullying prevention	−2.460	0.014
Confidence bullying prevention	−1.994	0.046
Familiarity bibliotherapy	−2.328	0.020
Confidence bibliotherapy	−1.292	0.196
Familiarity teaching empathy	−1.225	0.221
Confidence teaching empathy	−2.050	0.040

Qualitative Analysis All open-ended survey questions and anecdotal notes were analyzed using Corbin and Strauss's (2008) methods for open coding. We examined all written responses for themes related to the impact of the bibliotherapy experience on students and on teachers. We then created tentative labels that summarized participant experiences. Five major themes emerged: benefits of bibliotherapy for students, impact of bibliotherapy on student behavior, development of student empathy as a result of bibliotherapy, teacher confidence in bibliotherapy, and teacher desire to continue bibliotherapy. See Table 3.2.

Table 3.2 Categories, open codes, and associated concepts of bibliotherapy with students and teachers

Major categories	Open codes	Associated concepts
Students	Benefits of bibliotherapy for students	Expresses enjoyment Provides safe environment to explore topic Builds class community Helps relate to characters Emphasizes importance of topic Builds empathy
	Impact of bibliotherapy on student behavior	Helps bully to recognize actions Teaches strategies for prevention and intervention Encourages self-reflection Helps determine right/wrong actions Refers to characters and books when new situations occur Increases friendships and decreases instances of bullying Develops empathy
	Development of student empathy as a result of bibliotherapy	Compares situations, actions, and emotions to characters Discussions on perspective of others Relates to peers in different way Reasons what they should do by relating to character
Teachers	Confidence in bibliotherapy	Knows students know how to identify bullying Increases strategies for prevention and intervention Accesses resources for referral books and discussion guides Empowers to respond calmly and professionally
	Desire to continue bibliotherapy	Engages students Desires to implement throughout the year

Benefits of Bibliotherapy for Students As with any instructional strategy, value can often be determined in how students are positively impacted. Several teachers reported that the format of bibliotherapy, in this case interactive read-alouds, was a catalyst for student enjoyment. A second grade teacher wrote "My children love for me to read books to them and I feel like I have more of their attention when I read than any other time. It is the perfect avenue [to] discuss the topic [bullying]." Others discussed that children felt safe to discuss the actions and emotions of a character rather than having to use personal experiences. Another second grade teacher said "Sometimes, children relate to a topic they have previously experienced...when introduced in a non-confrontational manner and they aren't involved in the specific situation." A kindergarten teacher noted a difference in classroom community, which was a common theme. She wrote:

> It has made them aware that bullying and teasing doesn't just affect one person it affects everyone involved. We also learned that our words can be just as harmful as using hands, feet etc. to hurt others. The read-alouds have helped create a more loving atmosphere amongst the students

Other teachers pointed to the fact that using literature signifies importance to students. One kindergarten teacher explains "It gives a different voice to the necessity of standing up for what is right. Students know that if it is important enough to write about, then it is important enough to hear multiple times."

Impact of Bibliotherapy on Student Behavior Changing student behavior is an important aspect of any prevention program. Bibliotherapy can be used to help an antagonist to recognize the consequences of his actions. A kindergarten teacher noted this saying that one child with previous tendencies to bully had begun to notice her how her words were hurting others and had conferenced with the teacher about what she could do instead. A second grade teacher said that "friendships have blossomed" since beginning the intervention. A sixth grade teacher commented:

> There were some differences noted in one relationship among the higher level students. I think they identified with some of the situations in the books and realized they were being mean to this student. I have seen an acceptance of this formerly picked on student

The same teacher reported a decrease in the tendency of some students to laugh at inappropriate moments during reading and to choose other options over physical retaliation in the hallway. A fourth grade teacher conveyed "It [bibliotherapy] gets kids thinking about specific situations and gives them a chance to relate it to their own behavior as well as think of possible solutions." A teacher of a Comprehensive Disability Class (CDC) for students in grades 1–3 observed that she used bibliotherapy "to talk about empathy toward each other and read stories to recognize and build confidence to handle different situations." She also noted a decrease in the frequency of bullying behaviors in her classroom.

Development of Student Empathy as a Result of Bibliotherapy Louie (2005) wrote that empathy development might help students to "understand the perspectives, actions, and attitudes of the characters they encountered" (p. 567). We assert that students can transfer that to empathy for other students as well. A kindergarten teacher explained what this looks like in her classroom:

> The read-alouds were great for helping the students see what it feels like to be bullied or picked on through the character's eyes. It helped them to also know that it needs to be reported if and when you see someone being bullied or teased. I can tell a difference in some of my friends [sic.]behavior after the read-alouds

Another kindergarten teacher stated "The stories brought to life instances of bullying and it allowed them to see how people feel when someone either bullies another person or is willing to stand up to someone who is hurting you or another person." In addition to stepping into the shoes of a character to experience their emotions and thoughts, empathy can also be present as students compare their own situations and actions to others. A first grade teacher wrote:

> I have many students that will revert back to one of the books we have read and remind others not to act like the "Recess Queen", etc. They treat the characters in the book as if they were really students, the characters give them something a little more tangible to hold onto and I think this has been wonderful

Another teacher in first grade stated that she noticed her students developing rationale for their actions or future actions based on characters from the read-alouds, "we look for things that are the same about the situation". Many teachers reported that using bibliotherapy increased positive classroom interactions, which may be attributed to greater empathy for fellow students. A fourth grade teacher said that her students "…relate to each other in a different and more positive ways" after participating in the interactive read-alouds.

Teacher Confidence in Bibliotherapy For bibliotherapy to be a sustainable strategy, we have argued that it must fit into the existing curriculum. We also advocate that it must build teacher confidence in their abilities to identify, intervene, resolve, and prevent bullying behaviors. One sixth grade teacher addressed this in her comment, "[u]sing children's literature is a great confidence builder when it comes to decreasing the incidences of bullying among my students." Educators also pointed to the value of bibliotherapy for teaching and modeling strategies for both the bullied and bystanders. A first grade teacher said "I feel literature is a wonderful way to teach strategies for dealing with different situations." One sixth grade teacher reported that the use of bibliotherapy gave both her and her students "a larger menu" of "options" and strategies to both respond to and prevent bullying. Another first grade teacher continued "…I like how through discussions about incidents I have the background knowledge to point back to a book that we have read and take a moment to dissect what is going on and how we can solve the problem."

Teacher Desire to Continue Bibliotherapy While many teachers discussed activities that they were already implementing to address bullying behaviors, almost all were described as isolated activities occurring at the beginning of the year for community building and the establishment of class norms. Activities such as writing class manifestos, creating of class families, taping Crumpled Charlie back together after ripping a paper cut out while saying mean words, squeezing toothpaste to demonstrate that words and actions cannot be taken back, reviewing Tribes TLC agreements, and modeling with role play were described as events that occurred when school began. As our study neared the end of the school year, we were surprised to find that there was no evidence of ongoing bullying prevention activities beyond reminders of expectations and praising or disciplining behavior. This validated our hypothesis that there is a need for ongoing, year-round strategies such as bibliotherapy that can be easily implemented into the existing curriculum. One first grade teacher wrote "The read-aloud's [sic]were fantastic and I cannot wait to start the year out with these next year instead of reading them at the end of the school year." As one fourth grade teacher noted, "The children loved the books so I plan to search for more similar books to read to future classes throughout the school year." A sixth grade teacher also validated her plans for continuing bibliotherapy "[u]sing children's literature is a powerful way to teach many skills, including anti-bullying strategies."

Conclusions and Recommendations for Practical Application

With the many federal, state, and local mandates that school administrators and teachers must adhere to in our current school climate (Cox & Witko, 2011), we have identified bibliotherapy as a research-based strategy that fits within the existing curriculum while also encouraging bullying prevention (Enteman et al., 2005; Esch, 2008; Frey et al., 2005; Johnson et al., 2001; Rowan, 2007; Sullivan & Strang, 2002; Schechtman, 2006; Young & Ward, 2011). Most elementary and middle school classrooms already schedule a daily read-aloud time when teachers take 15–20 min to read books to students. This time is perfect for engaging with exemplary text through bibliotherapy using the six guidelines for implementation: motivation with introductory activities, reading time, incubation, follow-up discussion, evaluation and closure, and caregiver involvement. In our cautious quantitative analysis, we found that implementing bibliotherapy increased teachers' familiarity with bullying prevention methods, bibliotherapy strategies, and strategies to teach empathy as well as teachers' confidence in ability to prevent bullying. Qualitative analysis revealed that teachers perceived bibliotherapy to be beneficial for students, to impact their behavior, and to develop empathic behaviors. Teacher participants also reported both confidence in bibliotherapy for bullying prevention and a desire to continue the practice.

As we expand our research into bibliotherapy and bullying prevention, we intend to replicate the study using a larger population and focusing on outcomes of student behavior. We will also modify the timeline of delivery of supplies, such as trade books, until participants have submitted all pre-intervention data from pre-surveys and anecdotal notes. For future consideration, we suggest that it would be beneficial to find ways to tailor the use of exemplary text appropriate for bibliotherapy into readers' theater scripts with classrooms of school children. Additional studies would be warranted to measure the impact of readers' theater as bibliotherapy in both student behavior and teacher perception of bullying prevention.

Box 3.1 Where to Find Exemplary Text for Bibliotherapy

- *Database of Award-Winning Children's Literature* http://www.dawcl.com/
- With over 12,000 records from 142 award-winning books, readers can search by award category, age of intended audience, culture, format, genre, and more. Returned lists can be further narrowed down by selecting additional criteria. Brief annotated bibliographies are included.
- *The grown Up's guide to the best Children's books* http://www.best-childrens-books.com/childrens-books-about-bullying.html
- This site lists books from seven different sites and groups books based upon the number of other sites they are recommended on. For example, if a book is recommended on four sites, it will be listed in the grouping of books recommended on four other sites. If the book is recommended on three other sites, it is grouped with the books that are listed on three other bullying books sites, and so on. The site also includes lists for other children's issues such as disabilities, self-esteem, divorce, and death/dying.
- *Childhood Bibliotherapy database* http://childhoodbibliotherapy.blogspot.com/search/label/Bullying
- Though this site contains lists for a variety of topics, including bullying, it does mention some lesser known books that are worth a look. Also, it is broken into age categories, and some of the other topics border bullying, such as self-esteem, ethnic diversity, resolving conflicts, and dealing with differences, and might prove useful when dealing with the topic.
- *Book lists great stories with big heart* http://www.doinggoodtogether.org/bhf/read-together/
- While not a true bibliotherapy booklist, this website offers booklists at the primary picture book level and at the older chapter book level. At each level, it offers questions that either a teacher or a parent could discuss with students or with a child. The books are current. Educators and parents might also be able to use books from other categories, such as kindness, emotional awareness, diversity, homelessness, or poverty. There are links to a wealth of activities that a teacher could use to teach these concepts.
- *AFT Bullying Prevention Booklist for Students* http://www.aft.org/bullying-prevention-booklist-students
- From the webpage of the American Federation of Teachers comes a list of selections of books for bullying prevention. Each entry contains both an annotated bibliography and a link for purchasing. Texts are divided into three categories: children's/picture books, teens/preteens, and self-help for children. Additional links to bullying prevention resources are also provided at the bottom of the page and are categorized by general resources, those for parents, those for children, and other related resources.
- *Portrayals of bullying in Children's picture books and implications for Bibliotherapy* http://scholarworks.wmich.edu/cgi/viewcontent.cgi?article=1100&context=reading_horizons

- While not a website, this links to a study by Moulton, Heath, Prater, and Dyches that we adore. Of particular interest is the fact that the researchers looked at 38 books by age level, specific type of bullying, how the bullying was resolved, what the setting of the bullying was, if any adults were involved or not, and how bystanders were involved. Therefore, even just the chart from this study could prove useful to a classroom teacher searching for a specific scenario to meet the needs of his or her class as they vary from year to year.

References

Afolayan, J. A. (1992). Documentary perspective of bibliotherapy in education. *Reading Horizons*, 33, (2). Retrieved from http://scholarworks.wmich.edu/cgi/viewcontent.cgi?article=1498&context=reading_horizons

Bartle, L. R. (2016). *The database of award-winning children's literature*. Retrieved from: http://www.dawcl.com/

Beatty, W. K. (1962). A historical review of bibliotherapy. *Library Trends, 11*(2), 106–117.

Berthoud, E., & Elderkin, S. (2016a). *The novel cure: An A-Z of literary remedies*. Edinburgh, Scotland: Canongate Books.

Berthoud, E., & Elderkin, S. (2016b). *The story cure: An A-Z of books to keep kids happy, healthy, and wise*. Edinburgh, Scotland: Canongate Books.

Berthoud, E., & Elderkin, S. (2014). *The Novel Cure: From Abandonment to Zestlessness: 751 Books to Cure What Ails You*. Penguin Publishing Group: London, England.

Corbin, J., & Strauss, A. (2008). *Basics of Qualitative Research: Techniques and Procedures for Developing Grounded Theory* (3rd ed). Thousand Oaks, CA: Sage.

Cox, J., & Witko, C. (2011). Accountability and the "Narrowing" of the Curriculum. In *State Politics and Policy Conference 2011*.

Doll, B., & Doll, C. (1997). *Bibliotherapy with young people*. Englewood, CO: Libraries Unlimited.

Dovey, C. (2015). Can reading make you happier? *The New Yorker*. Retrieved from http://www.newyorker.com/culture/cultural-comment/can-reading-make-you-happier.

Enteman, J., Murnen, T., & Hendricks, C. (2005). Victims, Bullies, and Bystanders in K-3 Literature. *Reading Teacher*, 59(4), 252–364.

Esch, G. (2008). Children's literature: Perceptions of bullying. *Childhood Education, 84*(6), 379–382.

Forgan, J. W. (2002). Using bibliotherapy to teach problem solving. *Intervention in School and Clinic. Austin, 38*(2), 75–83.

Frey, K. S., Hirschstein, M. K., Snell, J. L., Edstrom, L. V., MacKenzie, E. P., & Broderick, C. J. (2005). Reducing playground bullying and supporting beliefs: An experimental trial of the steps to respect program. *Developmental Psychology, 41*(3), 479–491.

Goleman, D. (1995). *Emotional intelligence: Why it can matter more than IQ for character, health, and lifelong achievement*. New York: Bantam Books.

Hinduja, S. & Patchin., J. (2016). "Cyberbullying by Gender" retrieved from https://www.cyberbullying.org/2016-cyberbullying-data

Johnson, C., Wan, G., Anistine Templeton, R., Graham, L, & Sattler, J. (2001). "Booking it" to peace: Bibliotherapy guidelines for teachers. *Academic Exchange Quarterly*, 5(3), 172–176.

Karges-Bone, L. (2015). *Bibliotherapy: Children's books that train the brain and jumpstart the heart*. Dayton, OH: Lorenz Educational Press.

Louie, B. (2005). Development of empathetic responses with multicultural literature. *Journal of Adolescent and Adult Literacy, 48*(7), 566–576.
Lyman, F. (1981). The Responsive Classroom Discussion. *Mainstreaming Digest* (109–113). College Park, MD: University of Maryland College of Education.
Marilyn A. Campbell, (2003). Prevention and Intervention for Anxiety Disorders in Children and Adolescents: A Whole School Approach. *Australian Journal of Guidance and Counselling* 13 (01):47–62
McCulliss, D. (2012). Bibliotherapy: Historical and research perspectives. *Journal of Poetry Therapy, 25*(1), 23–28.
McMillen, P. (2014). A therapeutic collaboration: The bibliotherapy education project at Oregon State University. *OLA Quarterly, 12*(2), 14–15.
Moulton, E., Heath, M. A., Prater, M. A., & Dyches, T. T. (2011). Portrayals of bullying in children's picture books and implications for bibliotherapy. *Reading Horizons, 51*(2), 119–148.
Murray, R., Shea, M., & Harlin, R. (2006). Teachers rate trade books for bullying and the bystander. In M. B. Sampson, S. Szabo, F. Falk-Ross, M. Foote, & P. E. Linder (Eds.), *Multiple literacies in the 21st centuries*. The College Reading Association: College Station, TX.
O'Neill, A. (2002). *The Recess Queen*. Scholastic Press: New York City, NY.
Ouzts, D. T. (1991). The emergence of bibliotherapy as a discipline. *Reading Horizons, 31*, 199–206.
Patchin, J. & Hinduja, S. (2016). Bullying today: *Bulletpoints and best practices*. Thousand Oaks, CA: Corwin Press.
Pardeck, J. (1986). *Books for early childhood: A developmental perspective*. Philadelphia, PA: Gordon and Breach.
Polacco, P. (2001). *Mr. Lincoln's Way*. New York, NY: Philomel Books.
Reed, J.G. (2015). *The library- "A healing place for the soul"* [Blog post]. Retrieved from https://mcallenlibraryblog.com/2015/06/24/the-library-a-healing-place-for-the-soul/
Rowan, L. (2007). Making classrooms bully-free zones: Practical suggestions for educators. *Kappa Delta Pi Record, 43*, 182–185.
Rubin, R. (1979). Uses of bibliotherapy in response to the 1070s. *Library Trends, 32*, 239–251.
Schrodes, C. (1950) *Bibliotherapy: A Theoretical and Clinical - experimental Study*, University of California.
Shechtman, Z. (2006). The contribution of bibliotherapy to the counseling of aggressive boys. *Psychotherapy Research, 16*, 631–636.
Schultheis, M., & Pavlik, R. (1977). *Classroom teacher's manual for bibliotherapy*. Fort Wayne IN: Institute for the Study of Bibliotherapy.
Sullivan, A. & Strang, H. (2002) Bibliotherapy in the Classroom: Using literature to promote the development of emotional intelligence. *Childhood Education, 79*(2), 74–80.
Thibault, M. (2003). *Children's literature promotes understanding [Online article from Learn NC]*. Retrieved from: http://www.learnnc.org/lp/pages/635
Thompson, C. (2009). *Bibliotherapy and anxiety levels of 5th graders*. Retrieved from http://search.proquest.com/docview/305070305?accountid=28833
Young, T. A., & Ward, B. A. (2011). Bullies in recent books for children and young adults. *Reading Horizons, 51*(1), 81–92. Retrieved from: http://scholarworks.wmich.edu/reading_horizons/vol51/iss1/7/
U.S. Department of Health and Human Services, 2014. "Laws and Policies" retrieved from https://www.stopbullying.gov/laws.index.html

Chapter 4
Coaching Teachers in Bullying Detection and Intervention

Catherine P. Bradshaw, Tracy E. Waasdorp, Elise T. Pas, Kristine E. Larson, and Stacy R. Johnson

Coaching Teachers in Detection and Intervention Related to Bullying

Bullying is the most common form of aggression experienced by school-aged youth; it is widespread and has far-reaching academic, mental health, and behavioral impacts on individual students as well as on the school climate (National Academies of Sciences, Engineering, and Medicine, 2016; Swearer, Espelage, Vaillancourt, & Hymel, 2010). Although some prevention programs show promising effects (Bradshaw, 2015), and nearly all states now require some type of mandated professional development for educators to address concerns related to bullying (Cornell & Limber, 2015), research shows that teachers still struggle to detect bullying and rarely implement effective strategies to respond to bullying when it is detected (Bradshaw, Sawyer, & O'Brennan, 2007; Demaray, Malecki, Secord, & Lyell, 2013). The classroom is a particularly important context for bullying prevention, as the vast majority of bullying occurs within the classroom, due in large part to the proportion of time spent in the classroom relative to other school settings (Bradshaw et al., 2007; Demaray et al., 2013). These issues are especially challenging in urban middle schools where the rates of peer victimization are higher and concerns for personal safety impede adult intervention (Bradshaw et al., 2007). Therefore, teachers need additional professional development and support in

C. P. Bradshaw (✉)
Curry School of Education, University of Virginia, Charlottesville, USA
e-mail: cpb8g@virginia.edu

T. E. Waasdorp · E. T. Pas · K. E. Larson · S. R. Johnson
Bloomberg School of Public Health, Johns Hopkins University, Baltimore, MD, USA

J. U. Gordon (ed.), *Bullying Prevention and Intervention at School*,
https://doi.org/10.1007/978-3-319-95414-1_4

preventing but also detecting bullying and effectively responding to mitigate the behavior and its subsequent effects (Reinke, Herman, & Sprick, 2011).

To address these gaps in classroom-based prevention programming, our team developed an innovative, collaborative, and data-informed coaching model called the Bullying Classroom Check-Up, to assist teachers in *preventing*, *detecting*, and *intervening* with bullying behaviors in the classroom (see logic model in Fig. 4.1 and graphic in the Appendix). Specifically, the Bullying Classroom Check-Up (BCCU) intends to prevent bullying through foundational classroom management that specifically integrates social-behavioral expectations, the identification of bullying behaviors in the classroom, and teachers' selection and implementation of strategies to address and intervene with these behaviors in real time. The BCCU leverages existing research-based approaches, most notably the Classroom Check-Up (CCU; Reinke, 2006; Reinke, Herman, & Sprick, 2011). The CCU (Reinke, 2006) is a tailored coaching model that incorporates motivational interviewing with coaching in a nonevaluative, data-driven fashion to facilitate changes in teachers' skills and behaviors. A mixed-reality teaching simulator called TeachLivE© (Dieker, Hynes, Hughes, & Smith, 2008) was integrated into the coaching process to provide teachers an opportunity to practice prevention, detection, and responsive strategies to address bullying in real time, with the ongoing guidance of their trained coach. The ultimate goal of the BCCU is to reduce bullying through an improved classroom environment, where teachers prevent, adequately detect, and respond with effective teacher intervention, thereby minimizing the exposure to and consequences for youth directly involved (e.g., victims, perpetrators) and indirectly involved (e.g., bystanders/witnesses). This, in turn, should also improve the broader school climate.

In this chapter, we provide a rationale for the development of the BCCU and describe the core components of the model, including the original CCU and TeachLivE© simulator. We then discuss how qualitative data were used to tailor these two approaches and integrate them to become the BCCU. We conclude with a summary of data recently collected regarding the feasibility and acceptability of the BCCU, which is currently being tested in a small-scale randomized controlled trial with approximately 80 middle school classroom teachers. The overarching goal of this chapter is to advance readers' understanding of the importance of the classroom setting and teacher practices in relation to the prevention of bullying before it happens and also to provide early intervention strategies to address bullying when it does occur.

Background and Rationale for the Bullying Classroom Check-Up

Although bullying is common, being either a victim or a bully has been linked with serious adverse effects on social-emotional well-being, academic achievement, and health for involved youth (e.g., Vaughn et al., 2010). Within the context of urban

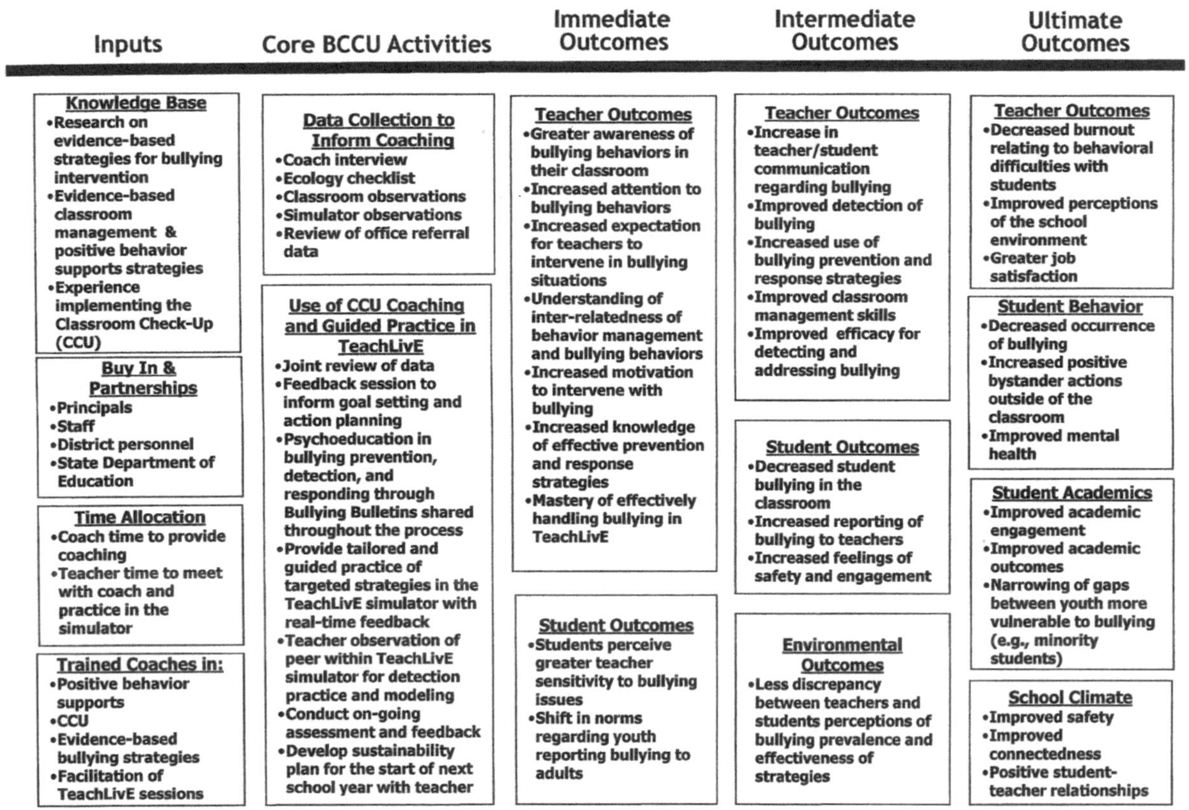

Fig. 4.1 Logic model for the bullying classroom check-up (BCCU)

schools, these negative impacts are further compounded by the common experience of multiple and chronic stressors, such as exposure to violence, decreased availability of resources, as well as academic, social, and emotional difficulties (e.g., Bradshaw, Rodgers, Ghandour, & Garbarino, 2009). In addition, racial and ethnic minority youth are at an increased risk for involvement in bullying as a victim, bully, or witness (Sawyer, Bradshaw, & O'Brennan, 2008).

The impact of bullying goes beyond the perpetrator and the victim, with studies showing that bullying negatively impacts those who witness bullying (i.e., bystanders) as well as the broader school climate (Lindstrom Johnson, Waasdorp, Debnam, & Bradshaw, 2013). For example, being bullied contributes to students' feeling fearful, which interferes with their ability to engage in learning (McDougall & Vaillancourt, 2015; Varjas, Henrich, & Meyers, 2009). Further, a high prevalence of bullying can create a norm within a school that bullying is acceptable behavior; students come to expect that it occurs regularly and do not respond in positive ways or seek assistance (Waasdorp, Pas, & O' Brennan, & Bradshaw, 2011). On the other hand, when teachers and other school staff proactively respond to bullying (e.g., effectively intervening), youth report feeling safer at school, report fewer instances of bullying, and report that they would respond more positively when they encounter bullying (e.g., by seeking adult assistance; Lindstrom Johnson et al., 2013; Waasdorp et al., 2011). As such, teachers are in an important position to prevent and intervene with bullying behaviors.

In fact, recent meta-analyses and reviews of bullying prevention programs concluded that prevention programs can produce meaningful impacts on bullying-related outcomes; in addition, these studies identified the use of consistent disciplinary methods and classroom management strategies, having classroom rules related to bullying, and training of teachers as core components of effective prevention programs (Bradshaw, 2013, 2015; Ttofi & Farrington, 2011). Aspects of the staff training, including the amount of time and the intensity of the training, were also positively associated with the efficacy of the programs (Farrington & Ttofi, 2009). These findings highlight the importance of prevention programming that focuses on training classroom teachers to effectively intervene and build a foundation for effective classroom management (Bradshaw, 2015). Moreover, students spend the majority of their time in classrooms, and thus it is not surprising that youth have more opportunities to experience bullying in the classroom than in other settings (Bradshaw et al., 2007). However, there has been less research on bullying prevention in diverse, urban settings, where rates of school violence are typically higher (Leff, Waasdorp, Waanders, & Paskewich, 2014); these issues are exacerbated by cultural norms that (1) discourage help-seeking and reporting of bullying to adults and (2) support aggressive retaliation (Lindstrom Johnson, Finigan, Bradshaw, Haynie, & Cheng, 2011).

Although teachers are in a key position to help curtail bullying behaviors, they often struggle to address bullying, in part due to their inability to detect it (Demaray et al., 2013), their inability to discriminate between typical peer interactions and subtle types of bullying behaviors (e.g., exclusion, rumor spreading, teasing; Bauman & Del Rio, 2006; Mishna & Alaggia, 2005), and their limited training on effective intervention and de-escalation techniques (Bradshaw, Waasdorp, O'Brennan, & Gulemetova, 2013; Hymel, McClure, Miller, Shumka, & Trach, 2015; Saarento, Garandeau, & Salmivalli, 2014). Many teachers expect that youth will resolve bullying conflicts on their own (e.g., Newman, 2003) and view non-physical aggression, such as verbal attacks and social exclusion, as less serious and easier for youth to cope with (Troop-Gordon & Ladd, 2015). Further, teachers underestimate both the prevalence of bullying and the negative impact it has on students at their school (Nicolaides, Toda, & Smith, 2002), which may in turn contribute to their lack of an adequate response to bullying. This is particularly concerning, given that targets of peer victimization are at a greater risk for social difficulties when their teachers do not show sensitivity to the seriousness of the behavior (Newman, Holden, & Delville, 2005; Yoon, Barton, & Taiariol, 2004). This may be especially true in middle schools, where students typically display a developmental shift, by decreasing the prevalence of physical aggression and increasing nonphysical (i.e., more covert) and electronic forms of bullying (Waasdorp, Horowitz-Johnson, & Leff, 2017), which are harder for teachers to detect (Bradshaw et al., 2007; Leff et al., 2014).

In fact, adults and students differ in their perception of the extent to which teachers effectively intervene in bullying situations, such that teachers typically believe they intervene in bullying situations more often than students report (Bradshaw et al., 2007; Waasdorp et al., 2011). Although teachers typically believe that their intervention is helpful, recent research indicates that the vast majority of students perceive that teachers actually make the situation worse when they intervene. This likely contributes to the low occurrence of students reporting bullying incidents to school staff; instead they tend to report bullying events to their friends and often ignore bullying situations or try to handle it themselves (Bradshaw et al., 2007; Waasdorp & Bradshaw, 2011). Effective classroom management has been shown to be critical for effective bullying prevention, with well-managed classrooms rated as having a more favorable climate, being safer and more supportive, and having lower rates of bullying and aggressive behavior (Bradshaw, 2013, 2015; Waasdorp, Bradshaw, & Leaf, 2012), and disproportionality (Bottiani et al., 2012).

This growing body of research illustrates how imperative it is to prepare teachers to prevent bullying but also to respond effectively to bullying when they witness it and when bullying is reported to them. Although professional development on bullying is common in schools, without coaching and ongoing support, it is unlikely that these efforts will impact behavior change (Pas, Bradshaw, & Cash, 2014). Moreover, while there is growing empirical support for the incorporation of individualized classroom coaching and guided practice for sustained improvements in teacher practices, there has been limited application of coaching to address bullying in classrooms (Pas et al., 2014). Explicit coaching on the prevention of, detection of, and intervention with bullying behaviors may promote the effectiveness of school-wide bullying initiatives, particularly in urban and diverse school settings where these aggressive behaviors can quickly escalate into violence. To address these gaps regarding the lack of classroom-based bullying prevention programming, we leveraged innovative technologies and approaches most commonly used to address behavior management and classroom instructional practices to target bullying behaviors specifically. In the next section, we summarize the core components of the BCCU, including the original CCU, as well as the TeachLivE© simulator, and relevant research supporting their inclusion in the BCCU model to prevent and intervene in bullying situations that occur in the classroom.

Core Components of the Bullying Classroom Check-Up (BCCU)

Classroom Check-Up The Classroom Check-Up (CCU; Reinke, 2006; Reinke, Herman, & Sprick, 2011) was originally developed as a classroom coaching model to provide support to teachers in classroom management (Reinke, Lewis-Palmer, & Merrell, 2008). The CCU was modeled after the evidence-based and rigorously tested Family Check-Up (Connell, Dishion, Yasui, & Kavanagh, 2007), a strategy shown to be effective with families of children with problematic behavior. The CCU aims to increase teachers' motivation to sustain classroom management and instructional practices that are identified as strengths during an assessment process, while providing coaching support to teachers in areas identified as relative weaknesses. More specifically, the CCU uses a combination of components that include a survey of the classroom's ecological factors, direct observation of the teacher, visual performance feedback (Reinke et al., 2008), and motivational interviewing (Miller & Rollnick, 2002; Reinke, Herman, & Sprick, 2011). Motivational interviewing is a communication approach used to minimize ambivalence about change and facilitate the teacher's motivation and self-guided change, rather than to direct it (Miller & Rollnick, 2002). Motivational interviewing has typically been used with individuals engaged in addiction or general psychiatric counseling, but the same principles have shown promise in increasing teachers' implementation of effective practices (Miller & Rollnick, 2002; Reinke et al., 2012). The CCU components are grounded in the social psychological literature and have collectively shown promise in changing teacher behavior and subsequently reducing problematic student behaviors (Reinke, 2006).

There are five steps to implementing the BCCU (see Fig. 4.2). Step (1) The coach assesses the classroom through the CCU motivational interview with the teacher, the use of a Classroom Ecology Checklist that the teacher completes, and classroom observations of teacher and student behaviors (see the original measures and tools in Reinke, Herman, & Sprick, 2011). The original CCU measures were adapted to address bullying. For example, the Ecology Checklist and Classroom Visit forms were adapted to include indicators relevant to bullying detection and intervention, and the interview has new sections about school policies related to bullying and the strategies the teacher uses to prevent and intervene with negative student interactions and bullying. Step (2) The coach provides integrated feedback drawing from the interview, self-report survey, and observational data, to identify both strengths and areas of need. The CCU process provides an objective and nonjudgmental vehi-

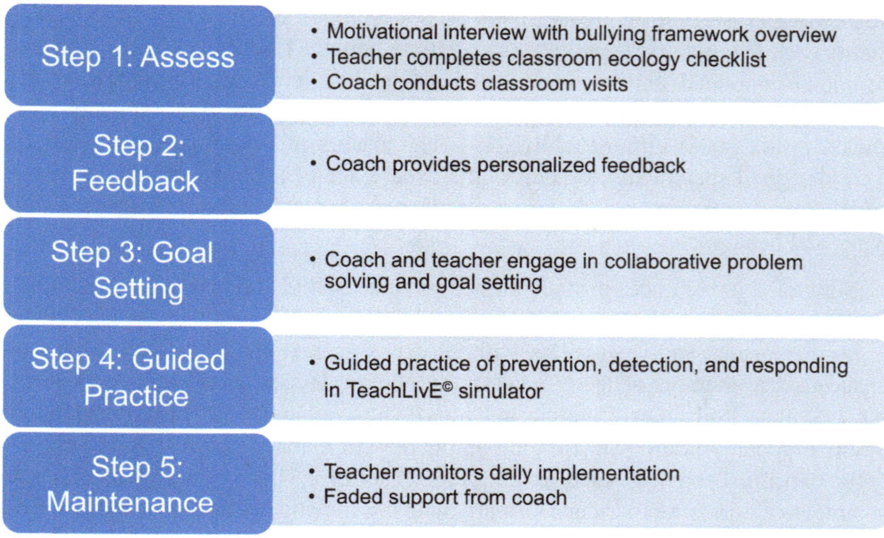

Fig. 4.2 The five steps of the Bullying Classroom Check-Up. (Adapted from Reinke et al. (2008) with permission)

cle for providing this feedback, which builds on the teacher's own reported motivations for change to promote acceptability and implementation of suggested interventions. The two main areas of feedback are positive behavior support related to classroom climate and social-emotional skills related to bullying prevention, detection, and responding. Step (3) Collaboratively, the teacher and coach develop an action plan for two goals, selecting from a set of strategies tailored to address bullying in the classroom. Step (4) The coach provides ongoing support via guided practice and performance feedback (Mesa, Lewis-Palmer, & Reinke, 2005) within the innovative TeachLivE© mixed-reality simulator. Using this technology, teachers interact with flexibly responsive avatars, which we elaborate on below. Step (5) Coach support is faded over time and eventually transitioned to the teacher, who self-monitors progress (Reinke, 2006). Although the BCCU model can be implemented over a single school year, a second year can also be included, whereby the coach continues to support the teacher through periodic check-ins on progress toward goals, conducting classroom visits, and providing additional coaching, modeling, and technical assistance to sustain progress or help set new goals.

The original CCU has been found to be effective as a means to increase behavior-specific praise given by teachers (Reinke et al., 2008), which in turn leads to a decrease in student disruptions. Teachers also reported favorable experiences with the CCU and found it to be effective, nonintrusive, and confidence evoking and to have social validity (Reinke et al., 2008). More recently, the CCU was adapted to increase teachers' use of culturally responsive practices in classrooms and similarly demonstrated improved teacher practices and acceptability (see Bradshaw et al., 2018; Pas, Larson et al., 2016).

TeachLivE© Simulator TeachLivE© was developed as an immersive, mixed-reality (i.e., part real, part synthetic) simulator where the teacher interfaces with five computer-generated, animated middle school-aged student avatars, who react to the human teacher in real time through a trained, live voice actor (i.e., interactor; see Dieker et al., 2008; http://teachlive.org). The avatars in the simulated experience were designed specifically to address the experience of teaching in urban settings and therefore represent racially diverse students across the continuum of personality types and behaviors.

Simulated experiences provide guided practice that (1) allows for opportunities that may not otherwise be available in the classroom, (2) permits individualization to teacher needs, and (3) is done without exposing real students to the harms of unsuccessful attempts at using new skills (Dieker, Hynes, Stapleton, & Hughes, 2007; Dieker, Rodriguez, Lignugaris-Kraft, Hynes, & Hughes, 2014). This technology is especially helpful for training adults how to manage and respond to potentially harmful behaviors such as bullying. TeachLivE© is not scripted, rather it leverages true-to-life experience virtually with the students' behaviors and responses enacted by trained actors. It is also modifiable, allowing for the virtual students' behaviors to be tailored to teachers' responses as needed. For example, we can also ensure that the bullying occurs, standardize how many times it happens and what form it takes, thereby enabling us to also use the simulator for assessment purposes (Dieker et al., 2014).

In the BCCU, as noted above, teachers interact with the TeachLivE© avatars in the fourth step to practice detecting bullying and using intervention strategies, as well as more general preventive behavioral and classroom management skills. The teachers are brought into the simulator on four occasions, ideally in pairs, to practice the strategies identified in their goal. All teachers are given the opportunity to come to the simulator in pairs, and while watching their teacher colleague in the simulator, they too can practice detecting bullying by recording each instance of bullying that they observed. Each TeachLivE© session is conducted at the teachers' schools, using portable equipment (e.g., laptop, hotspot Internet connection, webcam, and projector). Specifically, during the session, each teacher practiced using a strategy (e.g., setting expectations regarding positive peer interactions) for approximately 10 min, after which he/she received immediate data-based feedback from the coach. Teachers also had the opportunity to watch a second teacher practice and receive feedback. Finally, each teacher had a second chance at practicing for another 5–10 min.

Prior research on TeachLivE© suggests that teachers quickly became comfortable in interacting with the avatars (Dieker et al., 2014; Elford, Carter, & Aronin, 2013). Moreover, teachers' use of targeted skills has been shown to increase significantly following just one or two TeachLivE© sessions. Furthermore, in a pre-post intervention study where TeachLivE© was combined with the CCU to support special educators of children with developmental disabilities, trained observers witnessed teachers' generalization of the skills learned in the simulator to their classrooms, which may have been related to the simultaneous observation of improved student outcomes (see Pas, Johnson et al., 2016).

Psychoeducational Component of the BCCU Embedded within the CCU and TeachLivE© steps, the teacher is provided with six tip sheets, called "Bullying Bulletins," which are distributed by the coach throughout the school year (see example in Appendix A). These teacher-friendly handouts are intended to provide supplemental information on the specific topics addressed in the coaching and to serve as concrete reminders of specific strategies they can employ in the classroom. Specifically, the bulletins covered the following topics: (1) introduction and framework (i.e., establishing the importance of addressing bullying in schools and the teachers' role in prevention, detection, and responding); (2) detection of bullying behavior; (3) prevention of bullying behavior; (4) responding to bullying behavior in the moment, in a quick, clear, and consistent manner and how to work with students individually; (5) leveraging social and emotional approaches in teachers' responses to bullying, including reflection on their own language use in the classroom (i.e., THINK; is it thoughtful, helpful, insightful, necessary, and kind?), the use of open-ended questions to students prior to formulating responses, the reflection of student feelings, and I-statements; and (6) starting the school year off right, which summarizes how to begin the school year in a positive and proactive way. These last two bulletins (numbers 5 and 6) are intended to be distributed in the second year of BCCU implementation to review core elements of the model and sustain implementation, but could be embedded into a 1-year coaching protocol.

Development, Feasibility, and Acceptability of the BCCU

Consistent with the ADDIE model of systematic instructional design (Dick & Carey, 1996), we iteratively analyzed, designed, developed, implemented, and evaluated the BCCU strategy. Specifically, we first conducted a series of focus groups with students and middle school teachers to inform the adaption of the CCU and the scenarios to be used in the simulator for teachers to detect bullying and to practice using effective strategies to address it. We then worked with six middle school teachers using a rapid prototyping approach, whereby we solicited continual feedback and made adjustments and refinements to the BCCU and its components in real time. Following this initial phase of iterative development, we created a manual that outlines the BCCU model, which is currently being implemented and tested in a small-scale randomized study. During the iterative development process of the BCCU, focus group data as well as data on feasibility and acceptability were collected; these findings are summarized below.

Focus Groups to Inform Development of the BCCU Focus groups with students and teachers separately addressed participants' perceptions of (1) how teachers and students respond to bullying, (2) effective strategies for handling bullying, (3) what students wished teachers knew or did in response to bullying, and (4) what teachers felt they needed to prevent and respond to bullying. The sample for the focus groups was drawn from two ethnically diverse suburban schools. Specifically, we conducted focus groups in three schools; we included 17 student participants (6 boys, 11 girls) in 4 groups and 16 teacher participants (1 man, 15 women) in 3 groups. Focus groups were led by two experienced facilitators who were accompanied by two experts in bullying research. Notes taken by the bullying expert during the focus groups were analyzed by the study team. As summarized below, the feedback from teachers focused on four general themes, whereas the student feedback focused on three general themes.

Teacher Theme 1: Time and Efficiency Teachers described that dealing with bullying was difficult because they have many other tasks and expectations. For example, one teacher said, "I have too many academic pressures to get sidetracked by bullying behaviors." Teachers largely perceived that the bullying often occurred outside of the classroom (e.g., saying that it *spills over* from other classrooms, the halls, the Internet, and community). They also reported that bullying situations were too complex to efficiently address saying, "Students are friends one day and engaging in bullying the next" and "It is difficult to track these relationships or determine when students are just teasing each other versus actually bullying each other."

Teacher Theme 2: Low Self-Efficacy to Handle Bullying Teachers noted that students do not see them as the person to talk to; for example, one teacher said, "Students keep us out of the loop until something escalates," and another said, "Some kids don't feel comfortable telling the teacher; they don't even give it a chance. They go straight to the behavioral specialist. We only find out when the parents are angry." Teachers also felt that they do not have sufficient expertise to intervene or felt it is not their job to handle issues related to bullying. For example, one teacher reported that "Sending the students involved to a guidance counselor or assistant principal to deal with the students is easier because they are trained to deal with that stuff." Teachers made statements that suggested they did not believe certain behaviors were in fact bullying or suggested that bullying is a normative experience by making statements such as "There is too much drama" and "All kids are like this" regarding bullying behaviors in their classrooms.

Teacher Theme 3: Importance of Classroom Management A few of the teachers made statements suggesting that they recognized a link between behavioral classroom management and the escalation of student behavior into aggression or bullying. For example, one teacher said, "A teacher cannot deal with bullying when there are classroom management issues… [there are those] chaotic classrooms where [the] teacher is playing whack a mole and cannot even see what else is happening." Another said, "When classroom management varies from class to class, that makes it a struggle for teachers." Teachers also talked about the link between how the broader school context is managed and the level of student bullying. For instance, teachers discussed poorly monitored entrances and halls as places that allow for bullying to escalate.

Teacher Theme 4: Broader Systemic Issues Finally, teachers identified systemic issues surrounding the reporting of bullying with statements concerning the writing of referrals, the documentation of bullying incidents requiring too much time and effort, or the procedures for any other responses being unclear. Some teachers also indicated that they have been told by administration to minimize referrals, for example, "Teachers' hands are tied because they are not really supposed to refer" and "Teachers are supposed to complete these [bullying forms], but there are some [in] leadership telling teachers to clear it with them first and so they don't feel they are 'allowed' to complete a bullying response form; and even if they write a referral, it gets filed as something else. They don't want those data to show." Finally, teachers reported that their administrators do not respond consistently or effectively, saying, "They avoid giving suspensions even in dangerous situations (like having a weapon, without proven intent)."

In general, teachers felt that they do not have the time to understand what they perceive to be complex and often ambiguous student social interactions, and therefore are likely not going to be effective at responding. All four of these teacher themes pointed to the need for a time-sensitive strategy that was easy to use in a consistent manner and allowed for ample early detection and prevention not requiring administrators to respond.

Three clear and consistent themes emerged from the student data. Some of these themes overlapped with what teachers said, whereas others highlighted new areas that could be addressed through the BCCU intervention.

Student Theme 1: Time and Efficacy Similar to what teachers reported, students recognized that teachers have time constraints stating, "Teachers are busy and don't have time to have 1-on-1 talks with you. They don't give you as much talking time as you need to talk; they don't have time to be helpful." In other words, students appeared to link teachers' lack of time to the ineffectiveness of teachers' responses. Repeatedly, students suggested that teachers did not effectively help stop bullying or, if they did, made it worse. For example, "The teacher will see the bullying and act like she didn't see anything"; or "[The teacher will be] giving warnings, but never punish; threatening to call a parent, but never calling"; or "[one teacher] would defend the victim by teasing the bully"; and, finally, "[Teacher's] tell the victim to just get over it." Students voiced concerns consistent with those expressed by researchers that it is detrimental to victims to force conflict resolution strategies or apologies (e.g., Bradshaw, 2015). One student stated, "When they try to make [the] bully and victim talk, it is not helpful." Finally, students also suggested that teachers misinterpret what is happening in saying, "Teachers don't know the difference between when we're playing [i.e., joking] and when we are not."

Student Theme 2: Teacher Apathy A common sentiment was that teachers do not "seem to care or understand" what students are going through. One student illustrated this by saying "When teachers say, 'sticks and stones will hurt my bones, but not words', they should stop saying that because it really does hurt; it does hurt my feelings." Students felt that teachers want to make sure bullying does not occur in or negatively impact their classroom; as one student stated, "Teachers will warn not to bring it into the classroom; they won't care if it happens in someone else's classroom or the hallway, or right outside [their] classroom… they just don't want you to bring it in"; however, one student noted that "Teachers don't care to get the real story." This sentiment did concur with teachers' statements that they felt pressed for time and therefore could not handle bullying and that they felt that other school staff, such as the guidance counselor, was better suited to handle bullying.

Student Theme 3: Student-Teacher Connectedness When asked what they wished teachers knew or did in response to bullying, students discussed the need for teachers to connect with and get to know students. For example, "Teachers need to understand the kids' relationships" and "Teachers try to make you feel better, but they don't understand how hard it is, how much it can hurt to be teased." Students described what the effective adults do for them, "[Teachers that stop bullying] talk to the person outside of the classroom" and "Don't ask a lot of questions, let you talk it out." They shared, "[I would like teachers to] talk to those involved for more than 3 min. Try to find out what had happened; the whole thing beginning to end." Another student similarly noted that "Good teachers will talk to you, ask what is going on."

Summary of BCCU Adaptations Based on Focus Group Findings Based on the focus group data, we determined that in order to meet the needs of teachers, they would be provided with clear and concrete strategies for responding to bullying in a time-efficient but empathic manner. The adaptations to the CCU focus on building better and more authentic relationships with students, with a strong emphasis on relationships so that students know that teachers do genuinely care, even if they are pressed for time. We hypothesized that through a more open relationship, students would be more willing to have a productive discussion concerning important bullying matters with teachers (Waasdorp & Bradshaw, 2011, 2018). The focus groups and piloting also clarified that many teachers utilize a behaviorally focused approach to intervening and responding to bullying (e.g., just trying to stop the behaviors from occurring). Through the BCCU, teachers learn to shift this focus and validate student emotions and experiences, take the perspective of the students, and model appropriate ways of dealing with social conflict. Importantly, the BCCU was developed to include both behavioral responses, as well as emotional and social strategies for addressing bullying.

The resultant logic model for the BCCU (see Fig. 4.1) focuses on guiding teachers to implement strategies to prevent, detect, and respond to bullying. For example, the first Bullying Bulletin covers strategies for bolstering student connectedness through improved teacher-student relationships. Specifically, the bulletin suggests using regular noncontingent positive interactions to demonstrate care, monitoring students, and acknowledging their emotional states (e.g., when they may be having a bad day or conflict with another student) and letting students know they are there to help or talk. Through the second bulletin, teachers learn strategies for *detecting* bullying behaviors; this is complemented through self-monitoring, guided practice, and a strong focus on classroom management strategies, which relate directly to the prevention of bullying behaviors. For example, coaches instruct teachers to collect data (i.e., on their own or with the coach) about bullying and see if there are patterns of when it occurs (e.g., transitions or certain activities) and increase monitoring or change the routine associated with this time. Teachers also learn how to provide opportunities for students to report bullying and help the teacher know when bullying is happening, such as having a box in the room where students can put anonymous notes regarding personal or witnessed bullying situations. Then, teachers are taught how to *prevent* bullying behaviors through setting and displaying clear expectations that specifically relate to social interactions in the classroom, formally teaching the expectations through lessons throughout the year, and reinforcing positive interactions and instruction. Teachers develop a deeper understanding of the importance of drawing attention to the occurrence of positive peer behaviors and explicitly labeling the specific positive interaction. Finally, two of the bulletins summarize strategies teacher can use to *respond* to bullying witnessed in their classroom in a feasible and time-sensitive way. Teachers learn some strategies for acknowledging that bullying situations are stressful, emotionally taxing, and often hard to cope with; teachers explicitly and verbally convey that they sincerely want to understand what happened but would like to do this outside of class time and in a private space so other students do not hear. Teachers are provided some sample language they can use to reflect these concerns to students; for example:

> I am sorry this happened, as it sounds like it is frustrating for both of you. I would really like to know more about what happened. Let's follow up during lunch [or after class] so I can talk separately to you both and better understand what happened and how I can help.

> I know he said he was 'only kidding,' but this sounds like bullying to me. I would feel hurt if someone said something like that to me. While I don't know the entire situation, I want to learn more about what happened and how we can stop it from happening again. Let's talk at the end of the day.

Quantitative Data on Feasibility and Acceptability of the BCCU We also collected data from 80 middle school teachers, half of which were randomized to receive the BCCU coaching and the other half served as control teachers. Trained coaches hired and supervised by the project team completed tracking logs of the activities conducted with each intervention teacher and the fidelity to the BCCU coaching model. Coaches and intervention teachers also completed ratings of the coach-teacher alliance (see Johnson, Pas, & Bradshaw, 2016). Descriptive analyses were conducted to summarize the dosage and adherence to the model as well as perceptions of working relationship and benefits of the intervention. On average, the entire BCCU process took 8.65 h (SD = 1.85 h) for each coach and intervention teacher dyad. This included an average of 3.88 h (SD = 0.84 h) of active face-to-face teacher time and 4.77 h (SD = 1.27 h) of additional coach time (e.g., observations and preparation). Nearly every component of the initial BCCU interview, feedback, action planning, and simulator were implemented with 100% fidelity (i.e., with all of the participating teachers); the lowest fidelity was in planning for the simulator during goal setting (i.e., completed fully for 57% of teachers) and for practicing prevention strategies in the simulator (i.e., completed fully with 78% of teachers). Coaches rated high degrees of comfort in the classroom-based coaching and lower comfort in the first simulator (i.e., high comfort for 38% of teachers) that improved to 62% and 65% in the subsequent two sessions. Similarly, 41% of teachers self-reported that they were often or always comfortable during the first simulator session, and 82% were comfortable in subsequent sessions. Further, teachers reported positive reactions to the coaching (e.g., 97.2% reported that the coach delivered support, recommendations, and technical assistance in a clear and concise manner, and 91.6% reported that the time spent working with the coach was effective and productive) and to the benefits they received (e.g., 94.5% reported that the coach helped build their capacity to implement evidence-based strategies; 91.7% reported that the coaching increased their comfort with addressing bullying in the classroom; 83.4% reported that the coach had a positive impact on their classroom; and 83.3% reported that their students benefitted from the work with the coach). Moreover, 80.6% reported that they increased their knowledge of strategies to *prevent* bullying; 83.3% reported an increase in their knowledge of strategies to *detect* bullying; and 86.1% reported an increase in their knowledge of strategies to *respond* to bullying.

Together, the quantitative data suggested that the dosage and ratings of coach-teacher alliance for the BCCU were nearly identical to those reported in a study merging the CCU with TeachLivE© but were more narrowly focused only on classroom management (see Pas, Johnson et al., 2016) and took slightly longer than a CCU adaptation not including guided practice (see Pas, Larson, Reinke, Herman, & Bradshaw, 2016). These data suggested that the CCU can be expanded to focus on bullying and still maintain feasibility, acceptability, and fidelity.

Conclusions and Implications

In summary, the BCCU was developed as an adaption to the original CCU coaching framework to include additional guided practice on prevention, detection, and responding to bullying using an innovative mixed-reality simulator called TeachLivE©; these two core elements of CCU coaching and guided practice in the simulator were combined with additional tools and resources, such as the Bullying Bulletins. The BCCU is unique from other bullying prevention programs in that it is fully teacher focused and is not a manualized intervention delivered to students. In addition, it promotes social-emotional learning capacities and helps teachers to acknowledge that they recognize the issues and are responsive to bullying, to avoid students perceiving that teachers "don't care." The BCCU also leverages data collected from coaches and teachers to tailor a set of goals and an action plan co-developed by the teacher and coach, which includes guided practice opportunities in the TeachLivE© simulator.

The findings on the BCCU summarized above add to the growing body of work demonstrating that the coaching approach and guided practice through simulation are acceptable and efficient (Pas, Johnson et al., 2016); we seek to further determine whether it is also efficacious for changing teacher practice, as burgeoning research suggests. Moreover, these findings highlight the importance of classrooms and teachers as proximal influences on bullying and an important target for bullying prevention efforts (Bradshaw, 2013, 2015). While these feasibility and acceptability data suggest that the BCCU is a promising approach for addressing bullying in classrooms, rigorous outcomes-focused research is currently underway; specifically, we are currently conducting an approximately 80 middle school teacher randomized controlled trial to test the impacts of the program on student and staff outcomes.

The BCCU is intended to be delivered over the course of either one or two school years. In fact, our experience with the BCCU model and other similar coaching frameworks suggests that the provision of a second year of "booster" or supplimental coaching supports, although at a lower dosage than in the first year, is helpful for sustaining implementation. The BCCU also could be augmented to further maximize its impact. For example, the BCCU could be embedded within school-wide efforts, like Positive Behavioral Interventions and Supports, and perhaps school-wide professional development, to achieve stronger, school-wide impacts on bullying and related behavioral and social-emotional outcomes (see Bradshaw, Waasdorp, & Leaf, 2012; Waasdorp et al., 2012). The simulator technology could also be used with students to address bullying. For example, similar to the use of the BCCU with teachers, bystander students could learn to identify different forms of bullying and intervene in bullying situations in a way that would effectively diffuse the situation (see Waasdorp & Bradshaw, 2018). In addition, the simulator could be used within the context of a multi-tiered intervention to help students who are chronically victimized develop other strategies to respond to bullying. Further research is needed to explore various applications of the BCCU and its components, which to date appear to be efficient, acceptable, and feasible for addressing bullying in the classroom.

Acknowledgments Funding for the writing of this work and the research on the Bullying Classroom Check-Up come from the National Institute of Justice (grant number 2015-CK-BX-0008). The authors would like to acknowledge Drs. Wendy Reinke, Keith Herman, and Dana Marchese for providing consultation on the adaptation of the Classroom Check-Up and Dr. Lisa Dieker for consultation regarding the use of the TeachLivE© simulator.

Appendix: Sample Bullying Bulletin

Bullying Bulletin

MDS[3]

Sheppard Pratt Health System

Johns Hopkins University

Maryland's Safe and Supportive Schools

Maryland State Department of Education

Everyone in a school, from the principal, support staff, teachers, and students, plays a critical role in addressing bullying and creating a positive school climate. But teachers are especially important. Teachers can prevent bullying by building positive relationships, maximizing student engagement, and minimizing unstructured time. This in turn creates an environment that reduces the opportunity for negative social interactions.

Teachers should also respond appropriately and quickly to bullying when it does occur in their classrooms and throughout the school. Additionally, teachers have the unique opportunity to model and shape students' positive social interactions since they work with students in large group settings. Teachers often know their students best since they spend so much time with them.

What is Bullying?

Bullying is any unwanted aggressive behavior(s) by another youth or group of youths that involves an observed or perceived power imbalance and is repeated multiple times or is highly likely to be repeated.

Gladden, Vivolo-Kantor, Hamburger, & Lumpkin, 2014

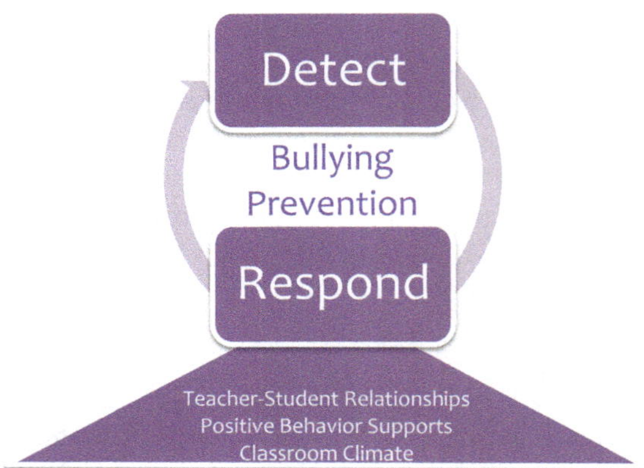

Talking to Your Students About Bullying

- Engage your students in discussions and role plays around bullying and strategies for responding
- Create a classroom definition and discuss the different forms of bullying (social/relational, verbal, physical, cyberbullying)
- Establish a system for students to communicate concerns and suggestions related to bullying, anonymously if needed

University of Virginia YOUTH-NEX Curry School of Education

Johns Hopkins Bloomberg School of Public Health

Starting Off the School Year to Prevent Bullying

Develop Relationships and Community

- Get to know your students: You can use an interest inventory or "learn about me" posters, which highlight the range of similarities and differences
- Encourage students getting to know one another: rotate assigned seats and mix up teams for group work
- Make yourself available: Encourage students to talk to you outside of class time and greet students in the hallway each day
- Seek student voice: Have a suggestion box; include students in the development of rules

Set up Clear Social Expectations

- Create 3-5 positively stated classroom rules that include social expectations, such as listening respectfully and kindly sharing different opinions
- Review relevant expectations at the start of class and new activities
- Review characteristics of being a positive group member and strategies to work together
- Reinforce expectations with behavior-specific praise

Use Effective Classroom Management

- Establish, communicate, and practice expectations and routines for *both* instructional and non-instructional time
- Reduce unstructured time by: 1) Using warm-up/drills to get class started, 2) Providing multiple opportunities for students to respond during class, 3) Using exit tickets at the end of class, 4) Providing options of "when you are finished" activities for students who finish tasks early
- Have structures in place to recognize students for exhibiting positive behaviors and provide consequences for students exhibiting inappropriate behavior

QUICK TIP: Review the MDS3 School Climate Survey data from last year to better understand the perceptions of bullying by students, teachers, & parents at your school.

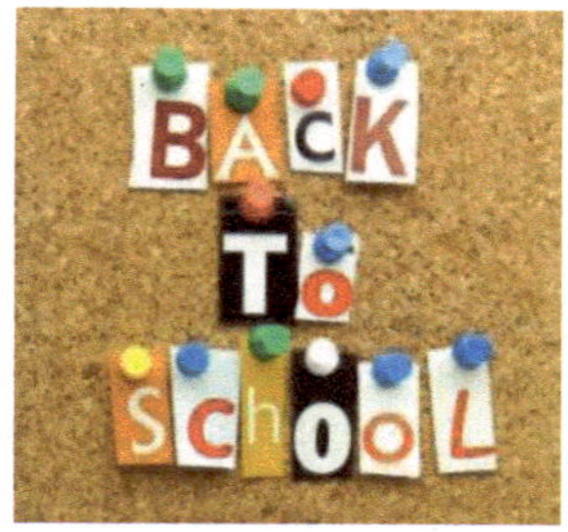

Responding to Bullying in Your Classroom and School

- When you see bullying: stop the situation immediately, label the behavior as bullying and harmful, remind of classroom expectations
- Examine the functions of the bullying or negative behaviors (e.g., attention seeking, avoidance of work)
- Consider skill deficits of all students involved such as poor problem solving, anger regulation, and social skills as contributors to the bullying or negative behavior
- Outside of class, problem solve strategies with the students to prevent the situation from reoccurring
- Don't forget to check in with the target(s) of the bullying to see how they are doing and remind them to use you as a trusted resource

References

Bauman, S., & Del Rio, A. (2006). Preservice teachers' responses to bullying scenarios: Comparing physical, verbal, and relational bullying. *Journal of Educational Psychology, 98*, 219–231. https://doi.org/10.1037/0022-0663.98.1.219

Bottiani, J. H., Bradshaw, C. P., Rosenberg, M. S., Hershfeldt, P. A., Pell, K. L., & Debnam, K. J. (2012). Applying double check to response to intervention: Culturally responsive practices for learning disabilities. *Insight on Learning Disabilities: Prevailing Theories to Validated Practices, 9*, 93–107.

Bradshaw, C. P. (2013). Preventing bullying through positive behavioral interventions and supports (PBIS): A multitiered approach to prevention and integration. *Theory Into Practice, 52*, 288–295. https://doi.org/10.1080/00405841.2013.829732

Bradshaw, C. P. (2015). Translating research to practice in bullying prevention. *American Psychologist, 70*, 322–332. https://doi.org/10.1037/a0039114

Bradshaw, C. P., Pas, E. T., Bottiani, J., Debnam, K. J., Reinke, W., Herman, K., & Rosenberg, M. S. (2018). Promoting cultural responsivity and student engagement through double check coaching of classroom teachers: An efficacy study. *School Psychology Review, 47*, 118–134. https://doi.org/10.17105/SPR-2017-0119.V47-2.

Bradshaw, C. P., Rodgers, C. R. R., Ghandour, L. A., & Garbarino, J. (2009). Social–cognitive mediators of the association between community violence exposure and aggressive behavior. *School Psychology Quarterly, 24*, 199–210. https://doi.org/10.1037/a0017362

Bradshaw, C. P., Sawyer, A. L., & O'Brennan, L. M. (2007). Bullying and peer victimization at school: Perceptual differences between students and school staff. *School Psychology Review, 36*, 361–382.

Bradshaw, C. P., Waasdorp, T. E., & Leaf, P. J. (2012). Effects of school-wide positive behavioral interventions and supports on child behavior problems. *Pediatrics, 130*(5), e1136–e1145. https://doi.org/10.1542/peds.2012-0243

Bradshaw, C. P., Waasdorp, T. E., O'Brennan, L., & Gulemetova, M. (2013). Teachers' and education support professionals' perspectives on bullying and prevention: Findings from a National Education Association (NEA) survey. *School Psychology Review, 42*, 280–297.

Connell, A., Dishion, T. J., Yasui, M., & Kavanagh, K. (2007). An adaptive approach to family intervention: Linking engagement in family-centered intervention to reductions in adolescent problem behavior. *Journal of Consulting and Clinical Psychology, 75*, 568–579. https://doi.org/10.1037/0022-006X.75.4.568

Cornell, D., & Limber, S. P. (2015). Law and policy on the concept of bullying at school. *American Psychologist, 70*, 333–343. https://doi.org/10.1037/a0038558

Demaray, M. K., Malecki, C. K., Secord, S. M., & Lyell, K. M. (2013). Agreement among students', teachers', and parents' perceptions of victimization by bullying. *Children and Youth Services Review, 35*, 2091–2100. https://doi.org/10.1016/j.childyouth.2013.10.018

Dick, W., & Carey, L. (1996). *The systematic Design of Instruction* (4th ed.). New York, NY: Harper Collins College Publishers.

Dieker, L., Hynes, M., Stapleton, C., & Hughes, C. (2007). Virtual classrooms: Star simulator. *New Learning Technology SALT, 4*, 1–22.

Dieker, L. A., Hynes, M. C., Hughes, C. E., & Smith, E. (2008). Implications of mixed reality and simulation technologies on special education and teacher preparation. *Focus on Exceptional Children, 40*(6), 1–20.

Dieker, L. A., Rodriguez, J. A., Lignugaris-Kraft, B., Hynes, M. C., & Hughes, C. E. (2014). The potential of simulated environments in teacher education: Current and future possibilities. *Teacher Education and Special Education, 37*, 21–33. https://doi.org/10.1177/0888406413512683

Elford, M., Carter, R. A., Jr., & Aronin, S. (2013). Virtual reality check: Teachers use bug-in-ear coaching to practice feedback techniques with student avatars. *Journal of Staff Development, 34*, 40–43.

Farrington, D. P., & Ttofi, M. M. (2009). School-based programs to reduce bullying and victimization. *Campbell Systematic Reviews, 6*, 1–149. https://doi.org/10.4073/csr.2009.6
Hymel, S., McClure, R., Miller, M., Shumka, E., & Trach, J. (2015). Addressing school bullying: Insights from theories of group processes. *Journal of Applied Developmental Psychology, 37*, 16–24. https://doi.org/10.1016/j.appdev.2014.11.008
Johnson, S., Pas, E., & Bradshaw, C. P. (2016). Understanding and measuring coach-teacher alliance: A glimpse inside the 'black box'. *Prevention Science, 17*(4), 439–449.
Leff, S., Waasdorp, T. E., Waanders, C., & Paskewich, B. (2014). Better understanding and intervening to prevent relational aggression. In M. D. Weist, N. A. Lever, C. P. Bradshaw, & J. S. Owens (Eds.), *Handbook of school mental health* (pp. 171–182). Boston, MA: Springer. https://doi.org/10.1007/978-1-4614-7624-5_13
Lindstrom Johnson, S., Waasdorp, T. E., Debnam, K., & Bradshaw, C. P. (2013). The role of bystander perceptions and school climate in influencing victims' responses to bullying: To retaliate or seek support? *Journal of Criminology, 2013*, 1–10. https://doi.org/10.1155/2013/780460
Lindstrom Johnson, S. R., Finigan, N. M., Bradshaw, C. P., Haynie, D. L., & Cheng, T. L. (2011). Examining the link between neighborhood context and parental messages to their adolescent children about violence. *Journal of Adolescent Health, 49*, 58–63. https://doi.org/10.1016/j.jadohealth.2010.10.014
McDougall, P., & Vaillancourt, T. (2015). Long-term adult outcomes of peer victimization in childhood and adolescence: Pathways to adjustment and maladjustment. *American Psychologist, 70*, 300–310. https://doi.org/10.1037/a0039174
Mesa, J., Lewis-Palmer, T., & Reinke, W. (2005). Providing teachers with performance feedback on praise to reduce student problem behavior. *Beyond Behavior, 15*, 3–7.
Miller, W., & Rollnick, S. (2002). *Motivational interviewing: Preparing people for change*. New York, NY: Guilford Press.
Mishna, F., & Alaggia, R. (2005). Weighing the risks: A child's decision to disclose peer victimization. *Children & Schools, 27*, 217–226. https://doi.org/10.1093/cs/27.4.217
National Academies of Sciences, Engineering, and Medicine. (2016). *Preventing bullying through science, policy, and practice*. Washington, DC: National Academies Press. https://doi.org/10.17226/23482
Newman, M. L., Holden, G. W., & Delville, Y. (2005). Isolation and the stress of being bullied. *Journal of Adolescence, 28*, 343–357. https://doi.org/10.1016/j.adolescence.2004.08.002
Newman, R. S. (2003). When elementary school student are harassed by peers: A self-regulative perspective on help seeking. *The Elementary School Journal, 103*, 339–355.
Nicolaides, S., Toda, Y., & Smith, P. K. (2002). Knowledge and attitudes about school bullying in trainee teachers. *British Journal of Educational Psychology, 72*(4), 105–118. https://doi.org/10.1348/000709902158793
Pas, E., Bradshaw, C., & Cash, A. (2014). Coaching classroom-based preventive interventions. In M. D. Weist, N. A. Lever, C. P. Bradshaw, & J. S. Owens (Eds.), *Handbook of school mental health* (pp. 255–267). New York, NY: Springer.
Pas, E. T., Johnson, S. R., Larson, K., Brandenburg, L., Church, R., & Bradshaw, C. P. (2016). Reducing behavior problems among students with autism Spectrum disorder: Coaching teachers in a mixed-reality setting. *Journal of Autism and Developmental Disorders, 46*(12), 3640–3652.
Pas, E. T., Larson, K., Reinke, W., Herman, K., & Bradshaw, C. P. (2016). Implementation and acceptability of an adapted classroom check-up coaching model to promote culturally responsive classroom management. *Education and Treatment of Children, 39*(4), 467–491.
Reinke, W. M. (2006). The classroom check-up: Advanced tools for effective coaching. In R. S. Sprick, J. Knight, W. M. Reinke, & T. McKale (Eds.), *Coaching for positive classrooms: Supporting teachers with classroom management* (pp. 139–167). Eugene, OR: Pacific Northwest Publishing.
Reinke, W. M., Herman, K. C., Darney, D., Pitchford, J., Becker, K., Domitrovich, C., & Ialongo, N. (2012). Using the classroom check-up model to support implementation of paths to pax.

Advances in School Mental Health Promotion, 5, 220–232. https://doi.org/10.1080/1754730X.2012.707441

Reinke, W. M., Herman, K. C., & Sprick, R. S. (2011). *Motivational interviewing for effective classroom management: The classroom check-up*. New York, NY: The Guilford Press.

Reinke, W. M., Lewis-Palmer, T., & Merrell, K. (2008). The classroom check-up: A classwide teacher consultation model for increasing praise and decreasing disruptive behavior. *School Psychology Review, 37*, 315–332.

Reinke, W. M., Stormont, M., Herman, K. C., Puri, R., & Goel, N. (2011). Supporting children's mental health in schools: Teacher perceptions of needs, roles, and barriers. *School Psychology Quarterly, 26*, 1–13. https://doi.org/10.1037/a0022714

Saarento, S., Garandeau, C. F., & Salmivalli, C. (2014). Classroom- and school-level contributions to bullying and victimization: A review. *Journal of Community & Applied Social Psychology, 25*, 204–218. https://doi.org/10.1002/casp.2207

Sawyer, A. L., Bradshaw, C. P., & O'Brennan, L. M. (2008). Examining ethnic, gender, and developmental differences in the way children report being a victim of 'bullying' on self-report measures. *Journal of Adolescent Health, 43*, 106–114. https://doi.org/10.1016/j.jadohealth.2007.12.01

Swearer, S. M., Espelage, D., Vaillancourt, T., & Hymel, S. (2010). What can be done about school bullying?: Linking research to educational practice. *Educational Researcher, 39*, 38–47. https://doi.org/10.3102/0013189X09357622

Troop-Gordon, W., & Ladd, G. W. (2015). Teachers' victimization-related beliefs and strategies: Associations with students' aggressive behavior and peer victimization. *Journal of Abnormal Child Psychology, 43*, 45–60. https://doi.org/10.1007/s10802-013-9840-y

Ttofi, M. M., & Farrington, D. P. (2011). Effectiveness of school-based programs to reduce bullying: A systematic and meta-analytic review. *Journal of Experimental Criminology, 7*, 27–56. https://doi.org/10.1007/s11292-010-9109-1

Varjas, K., Henrich, C. C., & Meyers, J. (2009). Urban middle school students' perceptions of bullying, cyberbullying, and school safety. *Journal of School Violence, 8*, 159–176. https://doi.org/10.1080/15388220802074165

Vaughn, M. G., Fu, Q., Bender, K., DeLisi, M., Beaver, K. M., Perron, B. E., & Howard, M. O. (2010). Psychiatric correlates of bullying in the United States: Findings from a national sample. *Psychiatric Quarterly, 81*, 183–195. https://doi.org/10.1007/s11126-010-9128-0

Waasdorp, T. E., & Bradshaw, C. P. (2011). Examining student responses to frequent bullying: A latent class approach. *Journal of Educational Psychology, 103*, 336–352. https://doi.org/10.1037/a0022747

Waasdorp, T. E., & Bradshaw, C. P. (2018). Examining variation in adolescent bystanders' responses to bullying. *School Psychology Review, 47*, 18–33. https://doi.org/10.17105/SPR-2017-0081.V47-1

Waasdorp, T. E., Bradshaw, C. P., & Leaf, P. J. (2012). The impact of schoolwide positive behavioral interventions and supports on bullying and peer rejection: A randomized controlled effectiveness trial. *Archives of Pediatrics and Adolescent Medicine, 166*, 149–156. https://doi.org/10.1001/archpediatrics.2011.755

Waasdorp, T. E., Horowitz-Johnson, Z., & Leff, S. S. (2017). Cyberbullying across the lifespan: Risk factors and consequences. In C. P. Bradshaw (Ed.), *Handbook of bullying prevention: A lifecourse perspective* (pp. 69–82). Washington, D.C: National Association of Social Workers (NASW) Press.

Waasdorp, T. E., Pas, E. T., O' Brennan, L. M., & Bradshaw, C. P. (2011). A multilevel perspective on the climate of bullying: Discrepancies among students, school staff, and parents. *Journal of School Violence, 10*, 115–132. https://doi.org/10.1080/15388220.2010.539164

Yoon, J. S., Barton, E., & Taiariol, J. (2004). Relational aggression in middle school: Educational implications of developmental research. *The Journal of Early Adolescence, 24*, 303–318. https://doi.org/10.1177/0272431604

Chapter 5
Cyberbullying Prevention and Intervention: Promising Approaches and Recommendations for Further Evaluation

Patricia Agatston and Susan Limber

Research on cyberbullying has increased dramatically since the early 2000s. Although studies on bullying among youth were first published in the 1970s (Olweus, 1973, 1978), research on cyberbullying did not appear in publication until 2004 (Brochado, Soares, & Fraga, 2017). Concerns about cyberbullying have grown as the involvement of children and youth with information and communication technologies (ICTs) has become commonplace. A recent report from the Center for the Digital Future (2017) found that 92% of American teens and adults used the Internet (up from 67% in 2000) and spent an average of 23.6 hours online per week (more than double the rate of 9.4 hours per week in 2000). Among teens, 92% report that they go online daily, including 24% who admit going online "almost constantly" (Lenhart, 2015). Although there are numerous benefits of ICT use, there are dangers as well, including cyberbullying. The purpose of this article is to review recent scholarship regarding the nature and prevalence of cyberbullying, its overlap with traditional forms of bullying, the costs of cyberbullying for those who are targeted, and promising and effective prevention and intervention strategies.

Cyberbullying Defined

Bullying among children and youth has been defined as "any unwanted aggressive behavior(s) by another youth or group of youths…that involves an observed or perceived power imbalance and is repeated multiple times or is highly likely to be repeated" (Gladden, Vivolo-Kantor, Hamburger, and Lumpkin (2014). This

P. Agatston (✉)
Prevention/Intervention Center, Cobb County School District, Marietta, GA, USA

S. Limber
Institute on Family and Neighborhood Life, Psychology Department, Clemson University, Clemson, SC, USA

J. U. Gordon (ed.), *Bullying Prevention and Intervention at School*,
https://doi.org/10.1007/978-3-319-95414-1_5

definition, which is largely consistent with Olweus' (1993) early conceptualizations, includes three key components: (1) it involves purposeful unwanted aggressive behavior that (2) typically is repeated over time and (3) occurs in a relationship characterized by an imbalance of power (Olweus, 2013; Olweus & Limber, 2017). Although these criteria have been questioned and even rejected by some (Bauman, Underwood, & Card, 2013; Canty, Stubbe, Steers, & Collings, 2016), this definition has been widely used by researchers (Olweus, 2013; Olweus & Limber, 2017).

Definitions of cyberbullying have been largely based on those of traditional bullying (Kowalski, Limber, & Agatston, 2012; Thomas, Connor, & Scott, 2015). For example, Smith and colleagues (Smith et al. (2008) define cyberbullying as "an aggressive, intentional act carried out by a group or individual, using electronic forms of contact, repeatedly and over time against a victim who cannot easily defend him or herself" (p. 376). Some have questioned the extent to which the three defining criteria of bullying can be applied to cyberbullying (National Academies, 2016), and many have noted that there are aspects of these criteria (notably the power imbalance and the repetition) that must be understood somewhat differently when applied to cyberbullying (Kowalski et al., 2012; Olweus & Limber, 2017). For example, as Smith and colleagues (Smith, del Barrio, & Tokunaga 2013) note, an online power imbalance may be revealed "in terms of differences in technological know-how between perpetrator and victim, relative anonymity, social status, number of friends or marginalized group position" (p. 36). Similarly, the focus on the criterion of repetition may need to be on the number of peers who are reached with a negative message or image online or the length of time that a hurtful message or image can remain in cyberspace, rather than on the cyberbully's behavior, which may constitute a single act (Olweus & Limber, 2017). Cyberbullying may assume different forms (including posting or spreading hurtful comments or embarrassing videos, spreading rumors, or threatening to hurt someone) and involve varied technologies, such as text messages, emails, social media, instant messaging through cell phone apps or computers, online gaming or other websites, video chats, and traditional phone calls.

Prevalence of Cyberbullying

As Olweus and Limber (2017) recently noted in their critique of cyberbullying research, there is "a bewildering array of prevalence estimates of cyberbullying" (p. 140). Indeed, in a review of 159 studies of cyberbullying among adolescents published between 2004 and 2014, Brochado et al. (2017) reported that lifetime prevalence rates for being cyberbullied ranged from 5% to 65%, and the percentage of youth who have experienced cyberbullying during the last year ranged from 1% to 61%. Lifetime estimates of cyberbullying others ranged from 1% to 44%, and rates of cyberbullying others over the past year ranged from 3 to 39%. Finally, lifetime prevalence rates for both cyberbullying others and also being cyberbullied ranged from 5% to 64%. There likely are several reasons for this heterogeneity. First, much variability may be attributed to different lengths of the recall period (e.g., lifetime, last year, last 6 months, last month, or last week; Kowalski, Giumetti, Schroeder, & Lattanner, 2014; Olweus & Limber, 2017). Second, differences may stem from the use of dissimilar threshold values for classifying a response as cyberbullying (e.g., whether it happened once vs. several times or more often; Olweus & Limber, 2017). Third, as Olweus argues (2013); Olweus & Limber, 2017), much of the heterogeneity in prevalence rates may stem from the study of cyberbullying "in isolation" from traditional bullying and a failure to carefully define behaviors. For example, cyberbullying prevalence rates are likely to be lower (and arguably more accurate) if researchers use language and definitions of bullying that makes it clear to the respondent that the behaviors of interest are distinct from general aggressive acts online or traditional forms of bullying (Kowalski et al., 2014; Olweus & Limber, 2017).

Several large-scale studies provide insight into the prevalence with which children and youth are cyberbullied. In the USA, three nationally representative studies are conducted with some regularity that provide data on bullying and cyberbullying: (1) the School Supplement to the National Crime Victimization Survey (NCVS), (2) the Youth Risk Behavior Survey (YRBS), (3) the Health Behaviour in School-aged Children (HBSC) survey, and (4) the National Survey of Children's Exposure to Violence (NatSCEV II). In the most recent version of the NCVS that assessed cyberbullying, 7% of 12–18-year-olds indicated that another student had done one or more of the following to them during the 2013 school year: posted hurtful information about them on the Internet, purposely shared private information about them on the Internet, threatened or insulted them through instant messaging, threatened or insulted them through text messaging, threatened or insulted them through e-mail, threatened or insulted them while gaming, or excluded them online (Musu-Gillette, Zhang, Wang, Zhang, & Oudekerk, 2017). By way of comparison, 22% had been bullied at school during the 2013 school year. In the YRBS, 16% of the 14–18-year-olds who were surveyed reported that they had been electronically bullied during the 2015 school year, including being bullied through e-mail, chat rooms, instant messaging, websites, or texting, during the 12 months before the survey (Kann et al., 2016). In this same survey, 20% reported that they had been bullied on school property during the previous 12 months. The HBSC survey of 10–16-year-olds in the USA, which included a detailed definition of bullying (Olweus, 1993), revealed that in 2010, 28% had been bullied at school at least once in the past couple of months and 12% had been cyberbullied in the past couple of months using a computer or e-mail (Iannotti, 2013). The HBSC is the only one of the four nationally representative studies to assess rates of cyberbullying others. In 2010, 28% had bullied others at least once in the past couple of months, and 8% had cyberbullied others at least once using a computer or e-mail. A fourth nationally representative survey, the NatSCEV II (Finkelhor, Turner, Shattuck, & Hamby, 2015), found that 6% of children (5–17) had experienced Internet or cell phone harassment during the past year.

The prevalence of different forms of cyberbullying varies depending upon the current popularity of technology and the age and gender of youth. In a recent nationally representative sample of 12–17-year-old middle and high school students in the USA, the most common ways in which youth indicate they have been cyberbullied in the past 30 days were having mean or hurtful comments posted online, having rumors spread online, having mean names or comments spread online that have a sexual meaning, being threatened online or through a cell phone text, and having a mean or hurtful picture posted online (Hinduja & Patchin, 2016).

Trends Over Time

Although attention to cyberbullying has increased dramatically, the extent to which rates have changed in recent years is unclear, based on nationally representative samples of youth (National Academies, 2016). For example, whereas the NCVS showed a twofold increase in the percentage of youth who had been cyberbullied between 2007 and 2011, rates declined two percentage points between 2011 and 2013 (National Academies, 2016). The YRBS showed a decline of cyberbullying between 2011 and 2013 (16.2% to 14.8%), but no significant change between 2013 and 2015 (Kann et al., 2016), and the HBSC survey showed a decline in rates of cyberbullying between 2006 and 2010 (National Academies, 2016). Moreover, Olweus (2013) found no significant changes in rates with which students had been cyberbullied or cyberbullied others in large samples of children and youth from Norway (2006–2010) and the USA (2007–2010).

Overlap with Traditional Bullying

Although available evidence does not indicate that cyberbullying has increased dramatically in recent years, it is still worth investigating whether this "newer" form of bullying has resulted in a substantial number of new victims and perpetrators of bullying (Olweus, 2013). Stated differently, are children and youth who are involved in cyberbullying largely the same youth who are involved in traditional bullying, or are they a unique group? Although there is some divergence of opinion on this question (Kubiszewski, Fontaine, Potard, & Auzoult, 2015), most researchers agree that there is substantial overlap between involvement in cyberbullying and traditional forms of bullying (Kowalski et al., 2014; Kowalsk & Limber, 2013; Olweus, 2013; Olweus & Limber, 2017; Smith et al., 2008). In their meta-analysis, Kowalski et al. (2014) found strong associations between the perpetration of traditional bullying and cyberbullying ($r = 0.45$) and between cyber victimization and traditional victimization ($r = 0.40$). In his large-scale studies of youth in Norway and the USA, Olweus (2013) found that of those who had been cyberbullied, 88% of American students and 93% of Norwegian students had also been bullied in at least one "traditional" way. Similarly, among those American youth who had cyberbullied others, 88% of American students and 91% of Norwegian students had bullied others in at least one "traditional way." Thus, only about 10% of students involved in cyberbullying had not also been involved in traditional forms of bullying. Others have also noted substantial overlaps of 50% (Ybarra and Mitchell (2004) and even 90% (Salmivalli & Pöyhönen, 2012). Baldry and colleagues (Baldry, Farrington, & Sorrentino, 2016) examined overlaps in traditional and cyberbullying among four distinct groups of youth: bullies-only, victims-only, bully/victims (those who are bullied and also bully others), and youth not involved in bullying. They found a particularly high degree of overlap between cyberbully/victims (those who are bullied and also bully others) and traditional bully/victims and for those not involved in cyberbullying and traditional bullying. Given differences among studies with regard to the conceptualization of bullying and its measurement, it is not surprising that there is not unanimity of findings regarding the existence and extent of overlap between cyberbullying and traditional bullying. However, most agree that a substantial proportion of youth involved in cyberbullying are also involved in traditional forms of bullying (Olweus & Limber, 2017), which has implications for prevention and intervention efforts. Future research will be useful to further explore the extent of overlap among subgroups of children and youth.

Risk and Protective Factors for Involvement in Cyberbullying

Although involvement in traditional bullying appears to be the strongest predictor of involvement in cyberbullying (Chen, Ho, & Lwin, 2017; Guo, 2016; Kowalski et al., 2014), researchers have identified a wide variety of other significant risk and protective factors for the involvement of children and youth in cyberbullying, including demographic factors such as age, gender, and socioeconomic status; factors related to an individual's personality, beliefs, and behaviors; and peer-, family-, and school-related factors. Because several recent systematic reviews (Ang, 2015; Baldry et al., 2016; Kowalski, Limber, & McCord, 2018) and meta-analyses (Chen et al., 2017; Guo, 2016; Kowalski et al., 2014) have examined these risk and protective factors in some detail, they will not be reviewed here.

Possible Effects of Cyberbullying

Extensive research has documented that traditional forms of bullying can have serious negative effects on children and youth who are targeted, including internalizing problems such as depression and anxiety (Bogart et al., 2014; Bowes, Joinson, Wolke, & Lewis, 2015; Copeland, Wolke, Angold, & Costello, 2013; Olweus, 1993; Reijntjes, Kamphuis, Prinzie, & Telch, 2010; Ttofi, Farrington, Lösel, & Loeber, 2011), psychosomatic complaints (Gini & Pozzoli, 2013), and health (Bogart et al., 2014). Researchers have also reported short- and long-term negative effects of cyberbullying on youth, including increased depression and anxiety, higher suicidal ideation, lower self-esteem, and poor academic performance and poorer reported health (Juvonen & Gross, 2008; Kowalski & Limber, 2013). However, given the high degree of overlap between involvement in traditional forms of bullying and cyberbullying, the question arises whether cyberbullying has negative effects on youth above and beyond negative effects from traditional bullying (Olweus & Limber, 2017). A number of recent cross-sectional and longitudinal studies have examined this question, and their results are not entirely consistent.

Findings from a handful of cross-sectional studies have reported that cyber-victimization is related to emotional problems such as depression, anxiety, suicidal ideation, and low self-esteem, even after controlling for youths' experience of traditional bullying (Bonanno & Hymel, 2013; Campbell, Spears, Slee, Butler, & Kift, 2012; Giumetti & Kowalski, 2016; Kim, Colwell, Kata, Boyle, & Georgiades, 2017; Schultze-Krumbholz, 2016; Sjursø, Fandrem, & Roland, 2016; Wigderson & Lynch, 2013). However, the variance for which cyberbullying accounts was typically small (e.g., 1–4%, Giumetti & Kowalski, 2016). In addition, Wigderson and Lynch (2013) found that cybervictimization (but not relational or physical victimization) was negatively associated with self-reported GPA, and Giumetti and Kowalski (2016) found that cyberbullying significantly predicted poorer self-reported grades and poorer health, even after controlling for experiences with traditional bullying.

However, there is disagreement among the studies with respect to the strength of the association between negative outcomes and different forms of bullying victimization. Some studies have found that traditional forms of bullying have a greater negative effect than cybervictimization. For example, in their study of 15- and 16-year-olds, Sjursø et al. (2016) found that the association between traditional victimization and depression was stronger than the association between cybervictimization and depression. Similarly, in their study of students in grades 8–10, Bonanno and Hymel (2013) found that the association between social victimization and depression was the strongest, followed by verbal victimization and then cyber victimization. Other studies have led to quite different conclusions. Campbell et al. (2012) found that although the 6th–12th graders in their study perceived that they were more impacted by traditional forms of bullying than cyberbullying, those youth who were cyberbullied reported higher levels of depression, anxiety, and social difficulties, than those who were bullied through traditional means.

In addition to these cross-sectional studies, a number of longitudinal studies have examined whether being cyberbullied contributes to negative outcomes, after controlling for possible experiences of being bullied in traditional ways. Several studies suggest that it does (Cole et al., 2016; Machmutow, Perren, Sticca, & Alsaker, 2012). For example, in a 12-month longitudinal analysis with 8–13-year-olds, Cole et al. (2016) found that cybervictimization, over and above traditional victimization, predicted changes in depression and negative cognitions (e.g., "Most people are against me"). McCuddy and Esbensen (2017) found that over time, middle school youth who were cyberbullied showed a greater propensity for substance use and nonviolent delinquency compared to youth who were traditionally bullied. In their 6-month longitudinal study of 7th graders, Machmutow and colleagues (2012) found that cybervictimization was a risk factor for adolescent depression, above and beyond traditional bullying. They further found that close social support (e.g., talking with close friends) buffered the negative impact of being cyberbullied, while assertive reactions (e.g., contacting the aggressor) aggravated the negative impact.

Other longitudinal studies have produced mixed or nonsignificant findings, however. For example, in a short-term (6 weeks) prospective study of 14–18-year-olds, Landoll and colleagues (Landoll, La Greca, Lai, Chan, & Herge, 2015) found that cybervictimization had a unique effect (beyond traditional bullying) on anxiety but did not predict increased depression over time, after controlling for traditional victimization. In their 2-year longitudinal study, Hemphill and colleagues (Hemphill, Kotevski, & Heerde, 2015) found that after controlling for traditional bullying and individual, peer, family, and school risk factors, there were no associations between cybervictimization and later problem behavior or mental health problems for 9th graders in the sample, but cybervictimization among students in grade 10 was associated with a fourfold increase in the likelihood of depressive symptoms 1 year later. Finally, Salmivalli and colleagues (Salmivalli, Sainio, & Hodges, 2013) found that traditional victimization had a unique effect on increased levels of depression among elementary and middle school students over the course of 12 months, but cybervictimization did not. Additional research is needed to clarify the extent to which involvement in cyberbullying (apart from involvement in traditional bullying) is related to later internalizing problems, psychosomatic complaints, externalizing problems, and academic difficulties among children and youth.

Cyberbullying Prevention

Just as research on the nature, prevalence, and outcomes of cyberbullying has increased dramatically in recent years, so too has attention to the prevention of cyberbullying. In its groundbreaking report, *Preventing Bullying Through Science, Policy, and Practice*, The National Academies of Sciences, Engineering, and Medicine (2016) found that "the most likely effective bullying prevention programs are whole school, multicomponent programs that combine elements of universal and targeted programs (p. 235)." Research focused on cyberbullying prevention is relatively new but demonstrates that there have been many variations on approaches to prevent cyberbullying, ranging from universal bullying prevention programs (many of which tend to have limited or no specific elements targeting cyberbullying) to cyberbullying-only whole-school approaches and finally to Internet Safety Education (ISE) lessons that include cyberbullying. This section will review recent program evaluation research in the emerging field of cyberbullying prevention that looks at various approaches and their efficacy.

Universal Bullying Prevention Programs Demonstrating Cyberbullying Outcomes

Evaluations of several universal bullying prevention programs have been conducted that show a reduction in cyberbullying as well as in-person bullying. The KiVa program, from Finland, is both universal and targeted, as it includes classroom lessons, supportive activities between lessons such as computer games, and specific actions that are taken when bullying occurs (Williford et al., 2013). Although its primary focus is in-person bullying, it does include several activities that address cyberbullying through classroom lessons that provide examples of cyberbullying and having students discuss ways to respond to cyberbullying. An evaluation of the program in Finland, which used a randomized controlled trial and targeted both elementary and middle school youth (grades 4–9) found a significant intervention effect, with lower cyber victimization among the KiVa students, regardless of age or gender (Williford et al., 2013). The effect on cyber perpetration however was moderated by age. Students below the sample mean age (12.9 years) reported lower frequencies of cyberbullying others than students in the control condition. However, older students showed no effect. Thus, while the program does appear to be effective in addressing cyberbullying perpetration and victimization, the authors suggest that school-based anti-bullying programs incorporate additional components aimed specifically at cyberbullying to strengthen the effects and involve parents, since many cyberbullying incidents occur at home.

The ViSC Social Competence Program in Austria is designed to reduce aggression and bullying and increase social competencies in schools (Gradinger, Yanagida, Strohmeier, & Spiel, 2015). Using a Train-the-Trainer model, teachers are trained to recognize and respond to bullying as well as to implement preventive measures at the school and classroom level. Students are educated about bullying and design a project that encourages them to take responsibility for what occurs in their class and develop strategies to prevent aggressive behavior. An evaluation of the program, using a randomized controlled trial, examined the program's effectiveness after 1 year of implementation among Austrian students in grades 5–7 (Gradinger et al., 2015). The results demonstrated that the program was effective for both cybervictimization and perpetration while controlling for traditional aggression, traditional victimization, and age effects. In subgroup analyses, the program was affective for girls (for both cyberbullying and cybervictimization) and for boys with respect to cyberbullying, but not for cybervictimization of boys (Gradinger et al., 2015). A follow-up study found that the cyberbullying effects were sustained at 6-month follow-up (Gradinger, Yanagida, Strohmeier, & Spiel, 2016). These initial findings suggest that anti-bullying programs are useful in addressing cyberbullying despite a lack of specific program elements to address online bullying, likely because of the similar mechanisms between traditional and cyberbullying. However, Gradinger et al. (2015, 2016) noted that effects likely would be even stronger if elements to address cyberbullying were included in the program (Gradinger et al., 2016).

Although its focus is broader than bullying prevention, the Second Step Violence Prevention Program has also shown effectiveness in reducing bullying through a focus on social emotional learning (SEL) (Espelage, Low, Van Ryzin, Polanin, & Joshua, 2015). The Second Step Middle School Program is a universal classroom-based SEL curriculum comprised of 15 lessons for sixth grade and 13 lessons for grades 7 and 8 that target risk and protective factors related to aggression, violence, and substance abuse (Espelage, Low, Van Ryzin, et al., 2015). The lessons are taught weekly or semiweekly throughout the school year. The program was evaluated with a 2-year cluster randomized trial (Espelage, Low, Polanin, & Brown, 2015). While the study did not find direct effects on perpetration of aggressive behavior after 3 years of implementation, at 1-year follow-up, researchers found statistically significant decreases in bullying, cyberbullying, and homophobic name-calling perpetration for Second Step schools (Espelage, Low, Van Ryzin, et al., 2015).

Cyberbullying Prevention Program Evaluation Outcomes

There are a number of cyberbullying prevention programs that have been developed as stand-alone programs or are part of a general Internet safety approach. The results from the cyberbullying prevention programs have been mixed, and many of these studies have serious methodological limitations (Della Cioppa, O'Neil, & Craig, 2015). In addition, Jones, Mitchell, and Walsh (2014) performed a content analysis of Internet Safety Education (ISE) curricula and noted that many did not use effective educational strategies for prevention education such as "skill-based objectives, adequate dosage, and practice opportunities" (p. 5). They recommended that prevention programs focus on skill building over simplistic messaging for youth not to cyberbully or engage in other risky online behaviors. In addition, they called into question the practice of treating ISE as a stand-alone issue, since most online problems have offline counterparts that are rarely discussed during the lessons, thus making the case for including cyberbullying as part of existing bullying prevention efforts. The following examples are programs that have been evaluated and focus on cyberbullying prevention only.

The Tabby project (Threat Assessment of Bullying Behavior of Youngsters in Internet) is a short-term school-based intervention implemented in Greece in which middle school students viewed four videos that presented different forms of cyberbullying (Athanasiades, Kamariotis, Psalti, Baldry, & Sorrentino, 2015). Trained teachers engaged students in discussion afterward, which included guidance on the safe use of the Internet as well as the impact and legal consequences of cyberbullying. The intervention was assessed through an online questionnaire, which was administered as a pre- and post-assessment among youth in five schools. Students were randomly assigned to experimental or control group by school. Although the evaluation indicated that the intervention was easy to implement, the results were inconclusive, as there were no significant differences between the experimental and control group on their "TABBY Profile," which assessed their risk profile of being a victim or perpetrator of cyberbullying (based on the risk factors of excessive and risky Internet use, involvement in traditional and cyberbullying, and estimates of future involvement in cyberbullying) (Athanasiades et al., 2015).

Another study in Greece focused on a whole-school intervention on psychosocial risk factors associated with cyberbullying, namely, lack of empathy, moral disengagement, and social cognitive variables related to cyberbullying (e.g., attitudes toward engaging in cyberbullying, social norms, and behavioral expectations for cyberbullying) (Barkoukis, Lazuras, Ourda, & Tsorbatzoudis, 2016). A total of 355 high school students from 11 junior and senior high schools were randomly assigned to intervention and control groups by school. The intervention focused on awareness raising regarding cyberbullying policies and norms, negative effects of cyberbullying, the accuracy with which students perceived the prevalence of cyberbullying among their classmates, and enhancing whole-school prevention efforts. Messages were communicated through both printed materials and meetings with groups of students. The campaign lasted 8 weeks, and its effectiveness was evaluated by means of a pre- and post-survey, which was administered immediately after the intervention. Compared with students in the control group, those in the intervention group showed decreases in moral disengagement and less positive views of a hypothetical cyberbully prototype. On the other hand, no differences between intervention and control groups were found for students' self-reports of empathy, attitudes, perceptions of social norms, and situational self-efficacy (Barkoukis et al., 2016). The authors recommended further research on actual behavior outcomes and possible long-term effects, as this study examined only immediate effects of the program.

Media Heroes (Medienhelden) is a school-based cyberbullying prevention program developed in Germany that focuses on promoting empathy; increasing students' understanding of cyberbullying, Internet safety, and legal consequences of inappropriate online behavior; and promoting positive bystander behavior (Chaux, Velásquez, Schultze-Krumbholz, Scheithauer, & Velásquez, 2016). Intervention strategies include role plays, debate, cooperative learning, and student-parent presentations. Two versions of the program were developed: a long version with fifteen 45-min sessions and a short version with four 90-min sessions implemented on a single day. In an evaluation of the intervention, 35 classrooms of 11–17 year-olds from 5 schools in Berlin, Germany were randomly assigned to intervention or control conditions (Chaux et al., 2016). Although the focus of the program was cyberbullying, the study showed positive results in reducing students' self-reports of traditional bullying perpetration with the long and short versions of the intervention 6 months after the intervention ended; however, the effects were greater for the longer program. The longer version of the program also showed a reduction in self-reported cyberbullying perpetration, compared to classes in the control group. However, neither the short nor long version was shown to reduce cybervictimization or traditional victimization (Chaux et al., 2016). The authors noted that it is likely that interventions designed to prevent cyberbullying will also reduce traditional bullying, since the risk factors and dynamics are similar and the behaviors are closely related (Chaux et al., 2016). They emphasized that further research is needed to explore how cyber and traditional bullying prevention efforts may complement each other and suggested that a reasonable approach might be to take a holistic approach that targets different types of bullying at different grade levels based on developmental appropriateness (Chaux et al., 2016).

Cyber Friendly Schools (CFS) is a whole-school cyberbullying prevention program that targets parents, students, and educators and includes home-school resources, 8 h of classroom lessons and activities, involvement of student leaders, restorative practices, and policy support (Cross et al., 2016). The program was tested in a large 3-year randomized controlled study in Australia, targeting 8th and 9th graders in 35 schools that were randomly assigned to intervention or control conditions (Cross et al., 2016). The main outcome measures were students' involvement in cyberbullying victimization and perpetration, and they were assessed by an online survey at baseline, after 18 months of intervention (posttest 1), and 1 year later (posttest 2). Overall, the CFS program was associated with a small but significant reduction in the odds of cyberbullying victimization and cyber perpetration in experimental schools after 18 months. However, at posttest 2, the intervention did not impact the frequency or extent of cyberbullying victimization or perpetration among involved students. The authors noted that teacher implementation was poor, with only about one-third of the CFS program implemented by teachers (Cross et al., 2016). The peer leaders demonstrated a sense of agency, belonging, and competence as a result of their training and support, as evidenced by pre-and posttest questionnaires and a pre- and post-qualitative in-depth interview with at least one peer leader from each participating experimental school (Cross, Lester, Barnes, Cardoso, & Hadwen, 2015). The authors noted that to improve the impact of the cyberbullying prevention program, it may be "important to simultaneously nest this intervention in a school program that is adequately addressing offline bullying" (Cross et al., 2016, p. 176.)

ConRed is a school-based ISE and cyberbullying prevention program designed to prevent cyberbullying through expert consultation with the school's climate planning committee over a period of 3 months, eight training sessions with students, a parent session, and an awareness-raising campaign (Ortegaga-Ruiz, Del Ray, & Casas, 2012). The program was implemented and evaluated in three schools in Cordoba, Spain, over the course of 3 months, using a quasi-experimental study with 893 students ages 11–19. Experimental and control groups were drawn from the same schools. Authors reported that the level of cyberbullying decreased significantly for students in the treatment group but not the control group, with regard both to aggression and victimization (Ortegaga-Ruiz et al., 2012). The findings were limited by the short-term evaluation and possible contamination across conditions within the same school.

Prevention Programs Focusing on Both Bullying and Cyberbullying

Several studies have focused on the evaluation of prevention programs that address both in-person and online forms of bullying with fairly equal emphasis. The Cyberprogram 2.0 is a school-based prevention program implemented with adolescents aged 13–15 in Spain. The program utilizes 19 1-h teacher-led sessions carried out weekly during the school term, which focused on face-to-face bullying, cyberbullying, and social emotional learning (Garaigortdobil & Martínez-Valderrey, 2015). The intervention was evaluated in three schools using a quasi-experimental design, with 93 students randomly assigned to the intervention group and 83 to the control group (Garaigortdobil & Martínez-Valderrey, 2015). Researchers found significant reductions in self-reported bullying and cyberbullying perpetration and victimization-based self-report at the end of the school term, as well as increases in empathy. Effect sizes were small to moderate (Garaigortdobil & Martínez-Valderrey, 2015). These findings, while promising, were limited by the small sample size and the lack of follow-up assessment.

The No Trap! program is a school-based prevention program implemented in Italy that focuses on both online and in-person bullying behavior and makes use of peer educators (Meneseni, Nocentini, & Palladino, 2012). In the initial version of the program, students from two schools designed a website to provide peer-to-peer content on bullying and cyberbullying prevention. Trained peer educators answered questions posted by users and moderated discussions. Peer educators also provided a class lesson on bullying and cyberbullying prevention and developed a television program for a local network on bullying and cyberbullying. In the initial evaluation of the program, 236 adolescents (grades 9–13, ages 14–20) in Tuscany, Italy, were surveyed at baseline and 6 months later. The study used a quasi-experimental, design with two experimental groups (one exposed to awareness-raising efforts only and a second group of highly involved peer leaders) and a control group. The only significant program effect was for the male peer leaders, who reported decreases in their self-reported bullying of others over time (Meneseni et al., 2012). In a follow-up study involving 375 adolescents (grades 9–13) in four high schools in Tuscany, modifications were made to the program, including increased attention to the bystander's role in supporting targets of bullying and greater involvement of subject teachers in interactive activities focused on bullying and cyberbullying (Meneseni et al., 2012). Researchers found significant decreases over time in the experimental group compared to the control group with respect to cybervictimization, bullying others, and being bullied, but not cyberbullying others based on self-report after 5 months (Meneseni et al., 2012). Two additional studies examined the efficacy of the No Trap! program among students in 9th grade (ages 14–15), using a quasi-experimental design with nonrandom assignment of schools to intervention and control groups (Palladino, Nocentini, & Menesini, 2016). In the first, which involved 622 students from 8 high schools in Tuscany, researchers observed significant program effects after 6 months of intervention, with intervention groups showing significant decreases over time with regard to bullying others, being bullied, cyberbullying others, and cybervictimization. This reduction remained stable at 6-month follow-up. In a separate study involving 461 adolescents in 9th grade in 7 high schools in Lucca, Italy, researchers observed significant program effects for youth in the intervention compared to the control conditions over time for both boys and girls (Palladino et al., 2016).

The Olweus Bullying Prevention Program (OBPP) is a school-wide bullying prevention program that includes interventions at four levels: school-wide interventions, classroom interventions, individual interventions, and community interventions. In several large-scale studies in Norway and the USA, the OBPP has demonstrated effectiveness in reducing bullying perpetration and victimization, as well as improving students' perceptions of adults' responsiveness to addressing bullying (Limber, Olweus, Wang, Masiello, & Breivik, under review; Olweus & Limber, 2010). Although the OBPP addresses cyberbullying through several of its interventions (e.g., it is included in the survey of students and addressed in the training of staff and in the core materials for school staff), beginning in 2008/2009, the OBPP has included and incorporated an optional supplemental cyberbullying prevention curriculum for use during classroom meetings (eight lessons for students in grades 6–8 and five lessons for students in grades 3–6; Limber, Kowalski, & Agatston, 2008/2014; Limber, Kowalski, & Agatston, 2009/2014). The middle/high school curriculum incorporates the use of peer leaders and addresses positive uses of technology to address bullying. Efforts are currently underway to examine the effectiveness of the OBPP in reducing specific forms of bullying (including cyberbullying) among schools that have (and have not) elected to use the optional cyberbullying resources.

Recommended Strategies for Cyberbullying Prevention

The previous section highlighted various evaluation studies and provided some evidence that more comprehensive programs focusing on both in-person and online bullying may be more effective than stand-alone cyberbullying programs. This conclusion supports research reviewed above that found that involvement in traditional bullying was the strongest predictor of involvement in cyberbullying (Athanasiades, Baldry, Kamariotis, Kostouli, & Psalti, 2016, Baldry et al., 2016; Chen et al., 2017; Guo, 2016; Kowalski et al., 2014).

Research is undoubtedly still scant on the effectiveness of stand-alone cyberbullying prevention programs and programs that incorporate cyberbullying prevention as part of comprehensive bullying prevention effort. However, there has been sufficient research regarding in-person bullying for the National Academies of Sciences, Engineering, and Medicine (2016) to make recommendations regarding best practices in bullying prevention. These include using a multitiered approach, addressing the social environment of the school through efforts such as effective staff training and the establishment of consistent rules and policies for behavior, engaging and training parents and family members, and integrating prevention efforts with other existing programs and supports (National Academies, 2016). Due to the significant overlap between traditional and in-person bullying, it is important to incorporate such practices into our cyberbullying prevention efforts as well. The next section will address some "best practice" components from bullying prevention as they apply to cyberbullying prevention, as well as some promising approaches that warrant further attention.

A Multitiered Approach

Our previous review of the literature regarding cyberbullying prevention programs made a case for utilizing a whole-school approach and imbedding cyberbullying prevention within the prevention efforts that are already in place to address bullying, rather than treating cyberbullying as a separate concern. This makes sense both for efficacy and efficiency, as schools struggle under the weight of many different prevention programs. A unifying framework to prevention can allow for better use of time and resources. A multitiered approach leverages universal, selected, and indicated prevention interventions (National Academies, 2016). Universal elements are aimed at reducing risks and promoting skills for all students (e.g., class meetings that focus on helping students understand different forms of bullying and the harms they cause, improve communication skills, and learn strategies to respond to bullying). Selective interventions target youth who are at risk for being involved in bullying (e.g., social skills training for small groups of children) and indicated preventive interventions are designed for those who are already displaying bullying behavior or who have already been bullied (e. g., intensive individual and/or family supports and programs).

Staff Training and Intervention

Training of school staff is widely viewed as "an essential element of successful bullying prevention efforts" (National Academies, 2016, p. 200). Several studies have found that school staff report a lack of training in preventing and responding to cyberbullying (Williford, 2015) and admit that they may not handle cyberbullying appropriately. In addition, many noncertified staff (such as clerks, cafeteria workers, or administrative assistants) report less self-efficacy to intervene in cyberbullying than certified staff (Styron Jr, Bonner, Styron, Bridgeforth, & Martin, 2015; Williford, 2015). These findings suggest that all school staff, including noncertified staff would benefit from training in both bullying and cyberbullying prevention and response. Law enforcement support staff such as school resource officers (SROs) should also be included in this training. A recent study of SROs indicated that they preferred to intervene in cyberbullying through education and early intervention rather than through punitive approaches (Broll & Huey, 2015). In addition, social support and guidance from SROs regarding Internet use have been found to have a moderating effect on the harmful impacts of cyberbullying, suggesting that SROs have an important role to play in assisting school staff or by helping students respond to cyberbullying (Wright, 2016). Training may particularly be important to educate adults about those forms of cyberbullying that are particularly distressing and warrant immediate and sensitive intervention. Jones and colleagues (Jones, Mitchell, & Turner, 2015) found that the most distressing forms of online harassment incidents are those that last longer (a month or more), include mixed elements of both in-person and online aggression, and/or included bias and sexual harassment.

Policies that Address Bullying/Cyberbullying

As noted by the National Academies (2016), clear expectations for students' behavior across all school contexts are critical for the development of a healthy school climate, and "clear anti-bullying policies are essential elements of a successful schoolwide prevention effort" (p. 220). All states in the USA have passed laws requiring schools to develop policies against bullying and most also include cyberbullying or online harassment (Bullying and Cyberbullying Laws across America, n.d.). The European COST (Cooperative in Science and Technology) working group on cyberbullying (Valimaki et al., 2012) emphasized that there was a need for cyberbullying to be included explicitly in school anti-bullying policies as a way to model respect and tolerance and be clear that cyberbullying is not acceptable. However, research is needed to examine the effectiveness of such policies on students' attitudes and behaviors (National Academies, 2016).

Parental Involvement

As highlighted above, parents can play important roles in the prevention of cyberbullying as supportive confidents to youth and as monitors of their children's use of the Internet (Ang, 2015; Chang et al., 2015). Focus group research with primary-aged school children suggests that parental supervision of their Internet and mobile phone use is helpful in preventing cyberbullying (Monks, Mahdavi, & Rix, 2016). On the other hand, active mediation (i.e., discussing both positive and risky behavior online as well as steps to minimize risk) and other collaborative strategies such as co-use are more effective in facilitating communication between parents and adolescents than restrictive mediation (i.e., setting time limits and blocking or restricting content) (Ang, 2015; Elsaesser, Russell, Ohannessian, & Patton, 2017). Thus, developmentally appropriate parent training/education around effective communication regarding strategies to reduce risk of cyberbullying, monitoring of ICTs, and bystander intervention is likely an important component for whole-school bullying prevention programs.

Efforts to Support Improved Family Functioning

Family conflict and violence are risk factors for involvement in cyberbullying (Guo, 2016), while protective factors include parental attachment, warmth, and support (Ang, 2015; Baldry et al., 2016; Chen et al., 2017). Research suggests that youth are generally accepting of parental advisement and intervention around cyber aggression (Goldstein, 2015); however, youth are more likely to express a willingness to talk to parents regarding cyberbullying experiences when they perceive trust to be present in their relationships (Certna, Machackova, & Dedkova, 2015). Thus, interventions that help develop relationship skills within the family and teach youth to manage difficult family situations may help reduce online bullying and victimization.

Promising Approaches That Warrant Further Attention

Recent scholarship has also pointed to some promising approaches to consider including in comprehensive cyberbullying prevention programs. Such approaches include a focus on social norms, bystander intervention, and family conferencing. Although the involvement of peers in cyberbullying is less well understood than their role in more traditional forms of bullying, research suggests that peers can increase the risk of involvement in cyberbullying (e.g., association with antisocial peers; Baldry et al., 2016; Guo, 2016) and also provide protective influences (e.g., support from peers; Kowalski et al., 2014). Adolescents who think their friends will approve of their participation in cyberbullying are significantly more likely to engage in cyberbullying (Bastiaensens et al., 2016). Bastiaensens et al. (2016) suggested that norms related to cyberbullying can influence both bystander behavior and the behavior of youth to initiate cyberbullying and concluded that social norms may be an appropriate area to target with prevention strategies. In addition, because the use of family conferencing has been found to be helpful for victims of other forms of crime, Langos and Sarre (2015) argue that family conferencing could be an effective restorative justice approach to cyberbullying intervention. While family conferencing has provided positive outcomes for victims in other forms of crime, research is needed to determine whether, and under what circumstances, positive outcomes will transfer to family conferences that involve cyberbullying.

Conclusions

Research on cyberbullying has increased dramatically in recent years, providing important insights into its nature and prevalence. One of the most consistent findings is the significant overlap between youths' involvement in traditional forms of bullying. Because cyberbullied youth also commonly experience other forms of bullying, additional research is needed to understand the extent to which involvement in particular forms of cyberbullying may (or may not) contribute to negative outcomes, above and beyond those experienced by traditional forms of bullying. Other gaps in knowledge also remain, including the extent to which involvement in cyberbullying is increasing or decreasing among children and youth in recent years and the effectiveness of different prevention and intervention efforts to address cyberbullying. As noted in the recent review by the National Academies (2016), "There remains a dearth of intervention research on programs related to cyberbullying"

National Academies, 2016, p. 9). Available evidence suggests that a multitiered approach will be most effective, which addresses known risk and protective factors, and imbeds cyberbullying prevention within the prevention efforts that are already in place to address bullying and promote safe and caring school communities. Research is also needed to examine promising approaches that include a focus on social norms, bystander intervention, and family conferencing.

References

Ang, R. P. (2015). Adolescent cyberbullying: A review of characteristics, prevention and intervention strategies. *Aggression & Violent Behavior, 25*, 35–42. https://doi.org/10.1016/j.avb.2015.07.011

Athanasiades, C., Baldry, A. C., Kamariotis, T., Kostouli, M., & Psalti, A. (2016). The "net" of the internet: Risk factors for cyberbullying among secondary-school students in Greece. *European Journal on Criminal Policy and Research, 22*, 301–317.

Athanasiades, C., Kamariotis, H., Psalti, A., Baldry, A. C., & Sorrentino, A. (2015). Internet use and cyberbullying among adolescent students in Greece: The "Tabby" project. *Hellenic Journal of Psychology, 12*, 14–39.

Baldry, A. C., Farrington, D. P., & Sorrentino, A. (2016). Cyberbullying in youth: A pattern of disruptive behaviour. *Psicología Educativa, 22*(1), 19–26.

Barkoukis, V., Lazuras, L., Ourda, D., & Tsorbatzoudis, H. (2016). Tackling psychosocial risk factors for adolescent cyberbullying: Evidence from a school-based intervention. *Aggressive Behavior, 42*(2), 114–122. https://doi.org/10.1002/ab.21625

Bastiaensens, S., Pabian, S., Vandebosch, H., Poels, K., Van Cleemput, K., DeSmet, A., & De Bourdeaudhuij, I. (2016). From normative influence to social pressure: How relevant others affect whether bystanders join in cyberbullying. *Social Development, 25*(1), 193–211.

Bauman, M., Underwood, M. K., & Card, N. A. (2013). Definitions: Another perspective and a proposal for beginning with cyberaggression. In S. Bauman, J. Walker, & D. Cross (Eds.), *Principles of cyberbullying research: Definition, measures, and methods* (pp. 41–46). New York: Routledge.

Bogart, L. M., Elliott, M. N., Klein, D. J., Tortolero, S. R., Mrug, S., Peskin, M. F., ... Schuster, M. A. (2014). Peer victimization in fifth grade and health in tenth grade. *Pediatrics, 133*(3), 440–447.

Bonanno, R. A., & Hymel, S. (2013). Cyber bullying and internalizing difficulties: Above and beyond the impact of traditional forms of bullying. *Journal of Youth and Adolescence, 42*(5), 685–697.

Bowes, L., Joinson, C., Wolke, D., & Lewis, G. (2015). Peer victimisation during adolescence and its impact on depression in early adulthood: Prospective cohort study in the United Kingdom. *The BMJ, 350*, 1–9.

Brochado, S., Soares, S., & Fraga, S. (2017). A scoping review on studies of cyberbullying prevalence among adolescents. *Trauma, Violence, & Abuse, 18*(5), 523–531. https://doi.org/10.1177/1524838016641668

Broll, R., & Huey, L. (2015). 'Just being mean to somebody isn't a police matter': Police perspectives on policing cyberbullying. *Journal of School Violence, 14*(2), 155–176. https://doi.org/10.1080/15388220.2013.879367

Bullying and Cyberbullying Laws Across America. (n.d.). Retrieved from https://cyberbullying.org/bullying-laws

Campbell, M., Spears, B., Slee, P., Butler, D., & Kift, S. (2012). Victims' perceptions of traditional and cyberbullying, and the psychosocial correlates of their victimisation. *Emotional and Behavioural Difficulties, 17*(3–4), 389–401.

Canty, J., Stubbe, M., Steers, D., & Collings, S. (2016). The trouble with bullying: Deconstructing the Conventional definition of bullying for a child-centred investigation into children's use of social Media. *Children & Society, 30*(1), 48–58.

Center for the Digital Future. (2017). *2017 Digital future report: Surveying the digital future*. Los Angeles: Center for the Digital Future at USC Annenberg.

Certna, A., Machackova, H., & Dedkova, L. (2015). Whom to trust: The role of mediation and perceived harm in support-seeking by cyberbullying victims. *Children & Society, 30*, 265–277.

Chang, F. C., Chiu, C. H., Miao, N. F., Chen, P. H., Lee, C. M., Chiang, J. T., & Pan, Y. C. (2015). The relationship between parental mediation and Internet addiction among adolescents, and the association with cyberbullying and depression. *Comprehensive Psychiatry, 57*, 21–28.

Chaux, E., Velásquez, A. M., Schultze-Krumbholz, A., Scheithauer, H., & Velásquez, A. M. (2016). Effects of the cyberbullying prevention program media heroes (medienhelden) on traditional bullying. *Aggressive Behavior, 42*(2), 157–165. https://doi.org/10.1002/ab.21637

Chen, L., Ho, S. S., & Lwin, M. O. (2017). A meta-analysis of factors predicting cyberbullying perpetration and victimization: From the social cognitive and media effects approach. *New Media & Society, 19*(8), 1194–1213.

Cole, D. A., Zelkowitz, R. L., Nick, E., Martin, N. C., Roeder, K. M., Sinclair-McBride, K., & Spinelli, T. (2016). Longitudinal and incremental relation of cybervictimization to negative self-cognitions and depressive symptoms in young adolescents. *Journal of Abnormal Child Psychology, 44*(7), 1321–1332.

Copeland, W. E., Wolke, D., Angold, A., & Costello, E. J. (2013). Adult psychiatric outcomes of bullying and being bullied by peers in childhood and adolescence. *JAMA, 70*, 19–26.

Cross, D., Lester, L., Barnes, A., Cardoso, P., & Hadwen, K. (2015). If it's about me, why do it without me? Genuine student engagement in school cyberbullying education. *International Journal of Emotional Education, 7*(1), 35.

Cross, D., Shaw, T., Hadwen, K., Cardoso, P., Slee, P., Roberts, C., ... Barnes, A. (2016). Longitudinal impact of the Cyber Friendly Schools program on adolescents' cyberbullying behavior. *Aggressive Behavior, 42*(2), 166–180.

Della Cioppa, V., O'Neil, A., & Craig, W. (2015). Learning from traditional bullying interventions: A review of research on cyberbullying and best practice. *Aggression and Violent Behavior, 23*, 61–68.

Elsaesser, C., Russell, B., Ohannessian, C. M., & Patton, D. (2017). Parenting in a digital age: A review of parents' role in preventing adolescent cyberbullying. *Aggression and Violent Behavior, 35*, 62–72.

Espelage, D. L., Low, S., Polanin, J. R., & Brown, E. C. (2015). Clinical trial of Second Step© middle-school program: Impact on aggression & victimization. *Journal of Applied Developmental Psychology, 37*, 52–63.

Espelage, D. L., Low, S., Van Ryzin, M., Polanin, J. R., & Joshua, R. (2015). Clinical trial of second step middle school program: Impact on bullying, cyberbullying, homophobic teasing and sexual harassment perpetration. *School Psychology Review, 44*(4), 464–479.

Finkelhor, D., Turner, H. A., Shattuck, A., & Hamby, S. L. (2015). Prevalence of childhood exposure to violence, crime, and abuse: Results from the National Survey of Children's Exposure to Violence. *JAMA Pediatrics, 169*(8), 746–754.

Garaigortdobil, M., & Martínez-Valderrey, V. (2015). Effects of cyberprogram 2.0 on 'face-to-face' bullying, cyberbullying, and empathy. *Psicothema, 27*(1), 45–51. Retrieved from http://libproxy.clemson.edu/login?url=http://search.ebscohost.com/login.aspx?direct=true&db=psyh&AN=2015-03876-007

Gini, G., & Pozzoli, T. (2013). Bullied children and psychosomatic problems: A meta-analysis. *Pediatrics, 132*(4), 720–729.

Giumetti, G. W., & Kowalski, R. M. (2016). Cyberbullying matters: Examining the incremental impact of cyberbullying on outcomes above and beyond traditional bullying in North America. In R. Navarro, S. Yubero, & E. Larranga (Eds.), *Cyberbullying across the globe: Gender, family, and mental health* (pp. 117–130). New York: Springer.

Gladden, R. M., Vivolo-Kantor, A. M., Hamburger, M. E., & Lumpkin, C. D. (2014). *Bullying surveillance among youths: Uniform definitions for public health and recommended data elements, version 1.0*. Atlanta: Centers for Disease Control and Prevention.
Goldstein, S. E. (2015). Parental regulation of online behavior and cyberaggression: Adolescents experiences and perspectives. *Cyberpsychology: Journal of Psychosocial Research on Cyberspace, 9*(4), 2. https://doi.org/10.5817/cp2015-4-2
Gradinger, P., Yanagida, T., Strohmeier, D., & Spiel, C. (2015). Prevention of cyberbullying and cyber victimization: Evaluation of the ViSC Social Competence Program. *Journal of School Violence, 14*(1), 87–110.
Gradinger, P., Yanagida, T., Strohmeier, D., & Spiel, C. (2016). Effectiveness and sustainability of the ViSC social competence program to prevent cyberbullying and cyber-victimization: Class and individual level moderators. *Aggressive Behavior, 42*(2), 181–193. https://doi.org/10.1002/ab.21631
Guo, S. (2016). A meta-analysis of the predictors of cyberbullying perpetration and victimization. *Psychology in the Schools, 53*(4), 432–453.
Hemphill, S. A., Kotevski, A., & Heerde, J. A. (2015). Longitudinal associations between cyberbullying perpetration and victimization and problem behavior and mental health problems in young Australians. *International Journal of Public Health, 60*(2), 227–237.
Hinduja, S. & Patchin, J. (2016). 2016 cyberbullying data. Retrieved from: https://cyberbullying.org/2016-cyberbullying-data
Iannotti, R. J. (2013). *Health Behavior in School-Aged Children (HBSC), 2009–2010. ICPSR34792-v1*. Ann Arbor, MI: Inter-university Consortium for Political and Social Research. Available from:. https://doi.org/10.3886/ICPSR34792.v1
Jones, L. M., Mitchell, K. J., & Walsh, W. A. (2014). *A content analysis of youth internet safety programs: Are effective prevention strategies being used?* Durham, NH: Crimes Against Children Research Center (CCRC), University of New Hampshire.
Jones, L., Mitchell, K., & Turner, H. (2015). Victim reports of bystander reactions to in-person and online harassment: A national survey of adolescents. *Journal of Youth and Adolescence, 44*(12), 2308–2320. https://doi.org/10.1007/s10964-015-0342-9
Juvonen, J., & Gross, E. F. (2008). Extending the school grounds? Bullying experiences in cyber space. *Journal of School Health, 78*, 496–506.
Kann, L., McManus, T., Harris, W. A., Shanklin, S. L., Flint, K. H., Hawkins, J., et al. (2016). Youth risk behavior surveillance: United States, 2015. *Morbidity and Mortality Weekly Report Surveillance Summaries, 65*(6), 1–174.
Kim, S., Colwell, S. R., Kata, A., Boyle, M. H., & Georgiades, K. (2017). Cyberbullying victimization and adolescent mental health: Evidence of differential effects by sex and mental health problem type. *Journal of Youth and Adolescence, 47*(3), 661–672.
Kowalski, R. M., & Limber, S. P. (2013). Psychological, physical, and academic correlates of cyberbullying and traditional bullying. *Journal of Adolescent Health, 53*(1), S13–S20.
Kowalski, R. M., Giumetti, G. W., Schroeder, A. N., & Lattanner, M. R. (2014). Bullying in the digital age: A critical review and meta-analysis of cyberbullying research among youth. *Psychological Bulletin, 140*, 1073–1137.
Kowalski, R. M., Limber, S. P., & Agatston, P. W. (2012). *Cyber bullying: Bullying in the digital age* (2nd ed.). New York: Wiley/Blackwell.
Kowalski, R. M., Limber, S. P., & McCord, A. (2018). *A developmental approach to cyberbullying: Prevalence and protective factors*. Under review.
Kubiszewski, V., Fontaine, R., Potard, C., & Auzoult, L. (2015). Does cyberbullying overlap with school bullying when taking modality of involvement into account? *Computers in Human Behavior, 43*, 49–57.
Landoll, R. R., La Greca, A. M., Lai, B. S., Chan, S. F., & Herge, W. M. (2015). Cyber victimization by peers: Prospective associations with adolescent social anxiety and depressive symptoms. *Journal of Adolescence, 42*, 77–86.

Langos, C., & Sarre, R. (2015). Responding to cyberbullying: The case for family conferencing. *Deakin Law Review, 20*(2), 299–319.

Lenhart, A. (2015, August). Teens, social media & technology overview 2015. Pew Research Center. Retrieved from http://www.pewinternet.org/2015/04/09/teens-social-media-technology-2015/

Limber, S. P., Kowalski, R. M. & Agatston, P. W. (2008/2014); Limber, S. P., Agatston, P. W., & Kowalski, R. M. (2008). *Cyber bullying: A prevention curriculum for grades 6–12*. Center City, MN: Hazelden.

Limber, S. P., Kowalski, R. M. & Agatston, P. W. (2009/2014); Limber, S. P., Agatston, P. W., & Kowalski, R. M. (2008). *Cyber bullying: A prevention curriculum for grades 3–5*. Center City, MN: Hazelden.

Limber, S. P., Olweus, D., Wang, W., Masiello, M., & Breivik, K. (under review). *Evaluation of the Olweus Bullying Prevention Program: A large scale study of U.S. students in grades 3–11*. Unpublished manuscript.

Machmutow, K., Perren, S., Sticca, F., & Alsaker, F. D. (2012). Peer victimisation and depressive symptoms: can specific coping strategies buffer the negative impact of cybervictimisation? *Emotional and Behavioural Difficulties, 17*(3-4), 403–420.

McCuddy, T., & Esbensen, F. A. (2017). After the bell and into the night: The link between delinquency and traditional, cyber-, and dual-bullying victimization. *Journal of Research in Crime and Delinquency, 54*(3), 409–441.

Meneseni, E., Nocentini, A., & Palladino, B. (2012). Empowering students against bullying and cyberbullying: Evaluation of an Italian peer-led model. *International Journal of Conflict and Violence, 6*(2), 313–320.

Monks, C. P., Mahdavi, J., & Rix, K. (2016). The emergence of cyberbullying in childhood: Parent and teacher perspectives. *Psicología Educativa, 22*(1), 39–48.

Musu-Gillette, L., Zhang, A., Wang, K., Zhang, J., & Oudekerk, B.A. (2017). *Indicators of school crime and safety: 2016* (NCES 2017–064/NCJ 250650). National Center for Education Statistics, U.S. Department of Education, and Bureau of Justice Statistics, Office of Justice Programs, U.S. Department of Justice. Washington, DC.

National Academies of Sciences, Engineering and Medicine. (2016). *Preventing bullying through science, policy, and practice*. Washington, DC: The National Academies Press. https://doi.org/10.17226/23482

Olweus, D. (1973). *Hackkycklingar och o¨versittare: Forskning om skolmobbning*. Stockholm: Almqvist & Wiksell.

Olweus, D. (1978). *Aggression in the schools: Bullies and whipping boys*. Washington, DC: Hemisphere.

Olweus, D. (1993). *Bullying at school: What we know and what we can do*. New York: Blackwell.

Olweus, D. (2013). School bullying: Development and some important challenges. *Annual Review of Clinical Psychology, 9*, 751–780.

Olweus, D., & Limber, S. P. (2010). Bullying in school: Evaluation and dissemination of the Olweus Bullying Prevention Program. *American Journal of Orthopsychiatry, 80*, 124–134.

Olweus, D., & Limber, S. P. (2017). Some problems with cyberbullying research. *Current Opinion in Psychology, 19*, 239–143.

Ortegaga-Ruiz, R., Del Ray, R., & Casas, J. (2012). Knowing, building, and living together on internet and social networks: The ConRed cyberbullying prevention program. *International Journal of Conflict and Violence, 6*(2), 302–212.

Palladino, B. E., Nocentini, A., & Menesini, E. (2016). Evidence-based intervention against bullying and cyberbullying: Evaluation of the NoTrap! program in two independent trials. *Aggressive Behavior, 42*(2), 194–206. https://doi.org/10.1002/ab.21636

Reijntjes, A., Kamphuis, J. H., Prinzie, P., & Telch, M. J. (2010). Peer victimization and internalizing problems in children: A meta-analysis of longitudinal studies. *Child Abuse & Neglect, 34*(4), 244–252.

Salmivalli, C., & Pöyhönen, V. (2012). Cyberbullying in Finland. In Q. Li, D. Cross, & P. K. Smith (Eds.), *Cyberbullying in the global playground: Research from international perspectives* (pp. 57–72). London: Wiley.

Salmivalli, C., Sainio, M., & Hodges, E. V. (2013). Electronic victimization: Correlates, antecedents, and consequences among elementary and middle school students. *Journal of Clinical Child & Adolescent Psychology, 42*(4), 442–453.

Schultze-Krumbholz, A. (2016). Feeling cybervictims' pain-the effect of empathy training on cyberbullying. *Aggressive Behavior, 42*(2), 147–156. https://doi.org/10.1002/ab.21613

Sjursø, I. R., Fandrem, H., & Roland, E. (2016). Emotional problems in traditional and cyber victimization. *Journal of School Violence, 15*(1), 114–131.

Smith, P. K., Mahdavi, J., Carvalho, M., Fisher, S., Russell, S., & Tippett, N. (2008). Cyberbullying: Its nature and impact in secondary school pupils. *Journal of Child Psychology and Psychiatry, 49*(4), 376–385.

Smith, P., del Barrio, C., & Tokunaga, R. (2013). Definitions of bullying and cyberbullying: How useful are the terms? *Principles of Cyberbullying Research: Definitions, Measures, and Methodology*, 26–40.

Styron, R. A., Jr., Bonner, J. L., Styron, J. L., Bridgeforth, J., & Martin, C. (2015). Are teacher and principal candidates prepared to address student cyberbullying? *Journal of At-Risk Issues, 19*(1), 19–28.

Thomas, H. J., Connor, J. P., & Scott, J. G. (2015). Integrating traditional bullying and cyberbullying: Challenges of definition and measurement in adolescents–a review. *Educational Psychology Review, 27*(1), 135–152.

Ttofi, M. M., Farrington, D. P., Lösel, F., & Loeber, R. (2011). Do the victims of school bullies tend to become depressed later in life? A systematic review and meta-analysis of longitudinal studies. *Journal of Aggression, Conflict and Peace Research, 3*, 63–73.

Valimaki, M., Almeida, A., Cross, D., O'Moore, M., Berne, S., Deboutte, G., … Sygkollitou E. (2012). Guidelines for preventing cyber-bullying in the school environment: A review and recommendations. Working Group 3 of COST Action IS081. Retrieved from: https://sites.google.com/site/costis0801/guideline

Wigderson, S., & Lynch, M. (2013). Cyber-and traditional peer victimization: Unique relationships with adolescent well-being. *Psychology of Violence, 3*(4), 297.

Williford, A., Elledge, L. C., Boulton, A. J., DePaolis, K. J., Little, T. D., & Salmivalli, C. (2013). Effects of the KiVa antibullying program on cyberbullying and cybervictimization frequency among Finnish youth. *Journal of Clinical Child & Adolescent Psychology, 42*(6), 820–833.

Williford, A. (2015). Intervening in bullying: Differences across elementary school staff members in attitudes, perceptions and self-efficacy beliefs. *Children & Schools, 37*(3), 175–184. https://doi.org/10.1093/cs/cdv017

Wright, M. F. (2016). Cyber victimization and psychological adjustment difficulties among adolescents: The role of technology mediation and social support from school resource officers. *Policing: An International Journal of Police Strategies & Management, 39*(3), 536–550.

Ybarra, M. L., & Mitchell, K. J. (2004). Online aggressor/targets, aggressors, and targets: A comparison of associated youth characteristics. *Journal of Child Psychology and Psychiatry, 45*(7), 1308–1316.

Chapter 6
"Coping with Bullying" Program in Greek Secondary Schools: An Evaluation

Christina Roussi-Vergou, Eleni Andreou, Eleni Didaskalou, Phillip Slee, and Grace Skrzypiec

Introduction

In recent years, school bullying has been recognized as a serious and devastating problem in Greece and other educational systems, and much of the research efforts in this area have been devoted to implementing effective interventions for its elimination (Didaskalou, Roussi-Vergou, & Andreou, 2015; Psalti, 2012; Van Deur, 2011). Data on the coping strategies that children and teenagers use to deal with school bullying have proven useful in addressing this alarming problem and informed many of the key components of anti-bullying programs implemented in schools (Didaskalou, Skrzypiec, Andreou, & Slee, 2016; Skrzypiec, Slee, Roussi-Vergou, & Andreou, 2013). It has been well documented that the systematic use by young people of counterproductive strategies for handling harassing interactions among peers is likely to increase their chances of being exposed to chronic and systematic victimization (Kochenderfer & Ladd, 1997; Smith, Talamelli, Cowie, Naylor, & Chauhan, 2004). Accordingly, Kanetsuna, Smith, and Morita (2006) strongly argue that whether casual school bullying turns into a chronic problem, this largely depends on the strategies that students themselves use to deal with peer aggression. Further, Murray-Harvey and Slee (2007) demonstrated that, in addition to victimization, adolescents' students' reliance on ineffective coping approaches also impacts on their overall mental health.

C. Roussi-Vergou
University of Thessaly, Volos, Greece

E. Andreou
Department of Primary Education, University of Thessaly, Volos, Greece

E. Didaskalou (✉) · P. Slee · G. Skrzypiec
School of Education, Flinders University, Adelaide, Australia
e-mail: edidask@sed.uth.gr

J. U. Mofe Gordon (ed.), *Bullying Prevention and Intervention at School*,
https://doi.org/10.1007/978-3-319-95414-1_6

Within this conceptual framework, the present study describes the core components and reports on the outcomes of an anti-bullying program which emphasizes on students' coping skills and aims to equip them with optimal strategies to handle peer harassment and accordingly strengthen their emotional resilience to bullying. The intervention program was originally constructed and tested in Australian schools and then adapted and implemented in Greek high schools. The theoretical underpinnings of the program are analyzed below, followed by a description of its prime objectives, the methodological approaches used for its implementation in Greek high schools, and finally the data regarding its effectiveness.

Bullying Coping Strategies: Theoretical Background

The theoretical foundations of the intervention are drawn from research on the coping strategies that adolescents employ to deal with stressful situations, such as problems of aggression by peers, indicating that ineffective coping is likely to contribute to increased personal adversities and subsequent negative emotions (Skrzypiec, Slee, Murray-Harvey, & Pereira, 2011). Notwithstanding the fact that that there is no consensual theory regarding the prime components of child and adolescent coping, the dimensions that are most commonly used to categorize coping strategies include problem-focused versus emotion-focused coping, also referred to in the literature as approach versus avoidance or engagement versus disengagement coping (Newman, 2008). With respect to bullying, problem-focused or approach-oriented coping strategies are found to correlate with a diminished likelihood of repeated victimization, whereas avoidance and emotion-related approaches are likely to add to expanding the extension of victimization over time (Murray-Harvey & Slee, 2006). Effective coping encompasses strategies such as looking for social backing by telling a peer or friend about your suffering, nonchalance, or opting to respond through an alternate way of acting. On the other hand, ineffective coping incorporates approaches like denying the existence of an incident, externalizing coping (e.g., cursing at someone), or crying and running away (Skrzypiec, Slee, Murray-Harvey, & Pereira, 2011; Kanetsuna et al., 2006).

A recent study conducted on a sample of Greek adolescent students revealed a significant correlation between the extent of their victimization and mindfulness about what they ought to do in order to prevent their harassment by peers (Didaskalou et al., 2015). As it was found, the students who were constantly bullied by their schoolmates were at the same time unaware about what they should do to assuage their peers' aggressiveness toward them. Frydenberg and colleagues (Frydenberg et al., 2004) argue that students are receptive and can successfully learn how to cope with stressful situations and adversities by using optimal strategies. Their theory is also applicable to the elimination of bullying in schools through the training of students in the implementation of effective coping strategies for dealing with aggressive interactions among peers (Terranova, 2009). The content of the program described below draws from the aforementioned views and emphasizes on learning and promoting optimal strategies especially for those students who are constantly victimized for ending their harassment by peers. A brief description of the main components of the program is provided below, followed by an analysis of the particular methodological procedure that were used for its adaptation and implementation in Greek high schools and the evaluation of its outcomes.

The Program "Coping with Bullying at School"

Content and Objectives

The core components of the program "coping with bullying at school" along with the delivery processes that were followed by the teachers involved in its implementation in Greek high schools have been drawn from and based on the well-known anti-bullying P.E.A.C.E. Pack intervention program (Slee, 1996). The program "coping with bullying at school" constitutes part of a wider holistic intervention scheme involving the entire school community that is being applied to Australian schools (P.E.A.C.E. Pack) (Skrzypiec, Slee, Murray-Harvey, & Pereira, 2011). The intervention program places emphasis on the victims' coping skills and aims to enhance the emotional resilience of students toward bullying. In particular, its main objectives are (a) to raise student awareness of the nature of bullying and its dynamics, (b) to provide students explicit training on optimal coping strategies, and (c) to evaluate the program's outcomes and the implementation of taught coping strategies. The program materials include (a) a DVD with four short films created by students recording incidents of physical bullying, social exclusion, verbal bullying, and electronic bullying; (b) workbook (for each student); (c) worksheets; and (d) instructions for the teachers assigned to its implementation. The central message of the entire program is "Stay Calm/Think Clearly." The program was delivered to students by their teachers in eight sessions. The teachers involved had received training on the process of its implementation and how to use the materials included in the program. The successful implementation of the program is linked to its continuous monitoring and making the most of the feedback from the involved students and teachers.

Methodological Procedures for the Program's Adaptation for Use in Greek Schools

The positive results from the implementation of the intervention program in Australian schools encouraged its adaptation and application to Greek secondary schools. This process was based on the established collaboration between researchers at the University of Thessaly and Flinders University in Australia (see Skrzypiec,

Roussi-Vergou, & Andreou, 2011). However, it is important to mention at this point that the Greek version of the intervention program concerns its implementation only at the level of the class and the evaluation of its outcomes accordingly.

As part of the process of the program's adaptation, its content and included materials were translated from English to Greek and vice versa, by a team of three researchers involved in studying school bullying and an English language teacher appointed in Greek high schools. For testing the program's adaptation, a pilot study was conducted during the academic year 2010–2011 (see Andreou et al., 2012). The program's implementation outcomes showed a remarkably similar picture regarding its effectiveness with the corresponding intervention outcomes in Australia. As expected, especially the students who were seriously bullied benefited from the program. The size effect of the intervention was estimated at $\eta^2 = 0.65$ (see Skrzypiec, Roussi-Vergou, & Andreou, 2011). These results were very encouraging for the wider implementation of the program in the schools of the province of Thessaly.

The Evaluation of the Program's Implementation in Greek High Schools

Research Aims and Questions

The purpose of this study was to evaluate the effectiveness of the intervention program, especially on coping strategies, through quantitative indicators. In particular, we aimed to collect data that answer the following research questions:

(a) *Was the anti-bullying program effective?*
We hypothesized that following the implementation of the program:

- The reported frequency of participant students' victimization will be reduced
- The reported perceived sense of safety of participants in school will be enhanced
- The reported self-efficacy of participants in coping with bullying will increase

(b) *Is there any change in the strategies that students use to counteract bullying, as a result of implementing the program? And if so, what are these specific strategies?*
We hypothesized that following the implementation of the program:

- An increase will be documented in the frequency of use by students of strategies that are considered effective (e.g., problem-centered or approach-oriented behaviors)
- A reduction will be observed in the frequency of use by participants of non-efficacious coping strategies (i.e., those involving the focus on feeling and avoidance)

Methodology

In order to evaluate the outcomes of the intervention program, an experimental approach was followed, which included a pre- and posttest assessment of the frequency of use of bullying strategies by the participant students. Accordingly, our sample consisted of participant students who received the intervention (intervention group) and participants who did not receive it (control group).

Participants

In our research participated a total of 932 students, attending 14 high schools in the province of Thessaly in Central Greece. Twelve out of the 14 high schools implemented the program (intervention group), while the rest two secondary schools participated only in the initial and recurrent measurements (as a control group). Among the participant students, 436 (46.8%) were boys and 425 (45.6%) girls, while 71 students did not report their gender (7.6%). Of the total sample, 667 students (71.6%) participated in the intervention group and 265 (28.4%) in the control group. Two hundred eight participants (208, i.e., 24.2%) had mother language other than Greek (23.9% for the intervention group and 24.8% for the control group, respectively). The students' age range was from 12 to 16 years old. The schools that were involved in this study prioritized the implementation of the program at year 7, and therefore over half of the participant students were between 12 and 13 years old (54.2%).

Measurements

For our measurements, we followed the proposed research protocol accompanying the intervention program. To assess the extent, the types of victimization experienced by participating students, as well as their perceived competence to handle victimization and the particular strategies they use, we asked them to fill in the questionnaire *"Living and learning at school: bullying at school"* (see also Skrzypiec, Slee, Murray-Harvey, & Pereira, 2011). The aforementioned questionnaire includes 68 items that aim to elicit information in relation to the following issues:

- *Demographic information of participant students* (e.g., gender, years of age, mother language other than Greek)
- *Frequency of reported student victimization.* The participant students were asked to report how often during the last month they had been bullied or threatened by one or more schoolmates. Students provided their answers in a Likert-type scale including six options ranging from every day to never

- *Types of victimization reported by students.* Those participants who reported that were victimized were then asked to indicate one or more of the suggested ways in which they were victimized or to report additional ways that were not included in the list. The suggested ones were hitting or kicking, calling nicknames, stealing personal belongings, cyber bullying, excluding, and ignoring (they do not speak to me)
- *Students' reported duration of exposure to victimization.* If participants reported having been victims during the past 3 months, they were then asked whether and how often they were victimized during the previous academic year. Students indicated their experiences in an eight-item scale ranging from 1 = I have not been victimized during the last year to 8 = more than 6 months
- *Students' perceived competence in coping with bullying (self-efficacy).* The perceived competence of participating students to counteract bullying was directly assessed. The students were asked to indicate on a Likert-type scale how well they manage to cope with school bullying. Students had to choose a value ranging from 1 = not very well to 7 = very well
- *Students' reported strategies for coping with bullying.* Participating students were asked if they had already used or would use one or more of the strategies included to cope with victimization at school. They were asked to indicate their responses on a five-point scale ranging from 1 = never to 5 = many times. For grouping the responses of students, a principal component analysis (PCA) was conducted in order to identify in a linear correlation the groupings of 43 variables related to coping strategies (Table 6.1). Initially, we calculated the Keizer-Meyer-Olkin index (KMO) to test the sample's sufficiency to be included in the analysis. The result of this calculation was the value "0.89" which is considered excellent as it approximates the "0.9" value. Also, the Bartlett's test of sphericity index was calculated in order to examine whether the correlations between the variables allow an analysis of factors to be conducted. This test gave $\chi^2 = 12{,}168.33$ (df = 903) which is statistically significant at the level $\alpha = 0.05$ ($p < 0.001$), indicating that the correlations in our data are suitable for inclusion in the analysis. Ten factors were removed with eigenvalues equal to or greater than "1″ that accounted for 56.3% of the total variance. Based on the grouping of strategies in the results of PCA, the Cronbach internal consistency index "α" was calculated. This was found to be satisfactory, and the groupings of the questions were coherent. Then, we summed up the individual scores in the questions of each factor to get a total score for each strategy

Data Collection Procedures and Analysis

The researchers contacted the principals of high schools as well as the directors of the health counseling centers of the province of Thessaly. Among the schools that indicated their interest in participating in this study, 12 accepted to implement the program and 2 more to serve as a control group for this study. The program was

Table 6.1 Summary of principal component analysis for the coping with bullying strategies

	Rotated factor loadings									
Items	1*	2*	3*	4*	5*	6*	7*	8*	9*	10*
55. Ask a teacher for help with the bullying	0.83									
28. Tell my parents/caregiver	0.80									
26. Tell a teacher	0.77									
65. Talk to my parents about the bullying	0.76									
64. Discuss the problem with a close family member (e.g., brother or sister or relative)	0.75									
56. Talk to a counselor about the bullying	0.73									
21. Ask an adult for help	0.71									
47. Use the school's anti-harassment/bullying procedures to deal with the bullying	0.63									
57. Get support from others, e.g., parents or friends	0.61									
52. Talk to a professional person outside the school	0.52									
41. Find others to spend time with	0.36									
29. Cry		0.80								
30. Look unhappy		0.79								
31. Look scared		0.75								
22. Get upset		0.73								
50. Help myself feel better by "letting off steam" (e.g., crying or screaming)		0.49								
39. Stay away from school to avoid the bullying		0.37								
51. Try to be cheerful despite the bullying			0.69							
53. Find a way to relax (e.g., play music, read, watch tv)			0.67							
38. Think of different ways I could solve the problem			0.49							
54. Keep fit and healthy so the bullying doesn't get me down too much			0.46							
42. Improve my relationship with the bully				0.83						
40. Try to make friends with the bully				0.83						
63. Show the bully that you are an OK sort of person				0.60						

(continued)

Table 6.1 (continued)

	Rotated factor loadings									
Items	1*	2*	3*	4*	5*	6*	7*	8*	9*	10*
23. Ask friends for help					0.69					
60. Use the school's peer support program					0.67					
61. Ask a friend to tell the bully to stop what they are doing					0.62					
37. Get other people's ideas for solving the problem					0.48					
45. Take my feelings out on others						0.86				
32. Take it out on someone or something else						0.81				
46. Make myself feel better by doing things that others wouldn't like me to do						0.44				
44. Hope that the bullying will sort itself out							0.65			
43. Wish a miracle would happen to stop the bullying							0.59			
49. See myself as being at fault							0.50			
20. Ignore the bullies								0.70		
25. Pretend it was not happening								0.65		
48. Avoid thinking about it								0.49		
33. Give in to the bullies								0.45		
62. Stick up for myself									0.54	
59. Fight back									0.52	
27. Get angry									0.50	
58. Tell the bully to stop what they are doing									0.41	
24. Get away from the bullies										0.59
% of variance	14.72	7.85	4.91	4.89	4.67	4.38	4.32	4.07	3.42	3.03
Cronbach's α	0.89	0.87	0.79	0.68	0.67	0.63	0.69	0.68	0.71	–
	1	2	3	4	5	6	7	8	9	10

*1. Seeking adults' support
*2. Emotional acting out and avoidance
*3. Optimism and positive attitude
*4. Becoming friends with bully
*5. Seeking peers' support
*6.Taking it out on others
*7.Wishful thinking
*8. Pretend as if not happening/submission
*9. Active defense
*10. Getting away

implemented in the form of an 8-week program, i.e., a session of 40–50 min duration was delivered to students each week in 8 consecutive weeks. In a typical academic year, the program started in schools around mid-October – when children completed the questionnaire on the first day of the program's implementation. We then advocated schools to complete the implementation of the program before the Christmas break – so that the second measurement can be taken immediately after the end of the holiday. Repetitive measurements were conducted 3 months after the last measurement and in any case by the end of April at the latest.

We analyzed the collected data using descriptive and inductive statistics. The first part of the analyses that were conducted concerned descriptive statistics and examined potential discrepancies among the participants on the basis of demographic variables such as gender, age, and language at home (other than Greek). The second part of the analysis focused on the extent to which intervention was effective and on which strategies were identified changes that could be attributed to the implementation of the program. To accomplish this, we conducted multivariate statistical analyses, a mixed ANOVA design, considering time (repeated measures) and condition according to the reported levels of initial exposure to victimization (Clark – Carter, 2004). Additionally, for examining the degree of correlation of victimization with specific strategies, we conducted a multivariate discriminant analysis by calculating the normal (canonical) multivariate correlation coefficients.

Results

Descriptive Statistics

Frequency of Exposure to Victimization

Valid responses were received from 849 of the 932 participants involved. With regard to the frequency of victimization, 1.5% reported that they were bullied daily, 2.8% most days of the week, 2% once or twice a week, 2.9% approximately once a week, and 22.6% less than once a week. 68.1% of the students reported that they had never been bullied.

The extent of exposure to bullying and victimization which students sustained has been recorded in three (3) categories: (a) those who were the recipients of severe victimization (ranging from incidences of bullying on a daily basis to being bullied once a week), (b) those enduring moderate victimization (exposed to bullying less than once a week), and (c) those who were unaffected by bullying (having never been bullied). The classification system showed that 9.3% of the participating children were identified as belonging to the category of those being severely victimized.

Table 6.2 Percentages of exposure to victimization according to students' gender

			Levels of victimization			Total
			Serious	Moderate	Safe	
Sex	*Boys*	*N*	53	109	269	431
		% within boys	12.3%	25.3%	62.4%	
	Girls	*N*	26	83	309	418
		% within girls	6.2%	19.9%	73.9%	
Total		N	79	192	578	849
		% Total	9.3%	22.6%	68.1%	100%

Table 6.3 Reported levels of victimization among students according to their mother tongue

			Levels of victimization		
			Serious	Moderate	Safe
Mother tongue spoken at home is other than Greek?	Yes	*N*	20	59	123
		% within "yes"	9.9%	29.2%	60.9%
	No	*N*	59	133	455
		% within "no"	9.1%	20.6%	70.3%

Gender Differences in the Frequency of Exposure to Bullying

With regard to the differences between boys and girls in terms of victimization rates, more boys reported that they were often seriously victimized (12.3% seriously intimidated), twice as many when compared to girls (6.2%) ($\chi 2$ = 15.32, df = 2, $p < 0.001$). Table 6.2 shows the rates of victimization for boys and girls.

Age Differences in the Rates of Victimization

According to Spearman's rho, there was no significant correlation (a = 0.05) between the ages of the students and their reported incidences of victimization. Given that victimization as a continuous variable does not follow any set distribution, a nonparametric test was selected as the most appropriate for the analysis.

Cultural Background Differences in the Frequency of Exposure to Intimidation

As shown in Table 6.3, pupils with a mother tongue other than Greek appear to experience more moderate rates of victimization than their counterparts of Greek origin. For children whose mother tongue is not Greek, the rates of exposure to victimization range from 9.9% for severely bullied to 29.2% for moderately victimized and 60.9% for unaffected students. For participants whose mother tongue is not

Greek, the respective reported rates of victimization were 9.1%, 20.6%, and 70.3%, respectively. The calculation of χ^2 revealed statistically significant differences ($\chi^2 = 7.21$, df = 2, $p < 0.05$) between the two aforementioned groups of participant students, possibly resulting from moderate exposure to bullying.

Types of Bullying

Name-calling was the most frequently reported bullying behavior (60.5%), followed by social exclusion "not being talked to" (37.9%), hitting and kicking (21.5%), removal of personal belongings (12%), and cyberbullying (9.6%). 30.9% of the students reported "other" forms of bullying to those included in the questionnaire. Incidences of hitting and kicking appear to be more prevalent among boys ($\chi^2 = 24.05$, df = 1, $p < 0.001$), whereas verbal exclusion (not being talked to) is more common among girls ($\chi^2 = 8.59$, df = 1, $p < 0.005$).

Previous Exposure to Victimization

The Spearman's rho ρ index points to a strong relationship between reported levels of victimization and previous exposure to bullying ($r = 0.53$, $p < 0.001$, 2-tailed).

Perceived Safety at School

It seems that most students feel safe at school with 55.66% reporting always, or almost always, feeling a sense of security, 30.7% feeling reasonably safe, 9.4% feeling safe only sometimes, and 4.3% never feeling safe. Chi-square (χ^2) revealed no differences related to gender, whereas those students with mother tongues other than Greek reported feeling less safe at school ($\chi^2 = 13.78$, df = 3, $p < 0.005$, 2-tailed). No differences related to age were noted.

Self-Efficacy in Coping with Bullying

Perceived efficacy in coping with victimization was assessed through responses given by students to the question of how well they managed to handle bullying. Figure 6.1 presents the distribution of their responses on a scale ranging from 1 = not very well to 7 = very well. The self-efficacy of students was negatively correlated with their levels of exposure to victimization (Spearman's rho = 0.45, $p < 0.001$, 2-tailed) and positively with their perceptions of safety at school (Spearman's rho = 0.48, $p < 0.001$, 2-tailed).

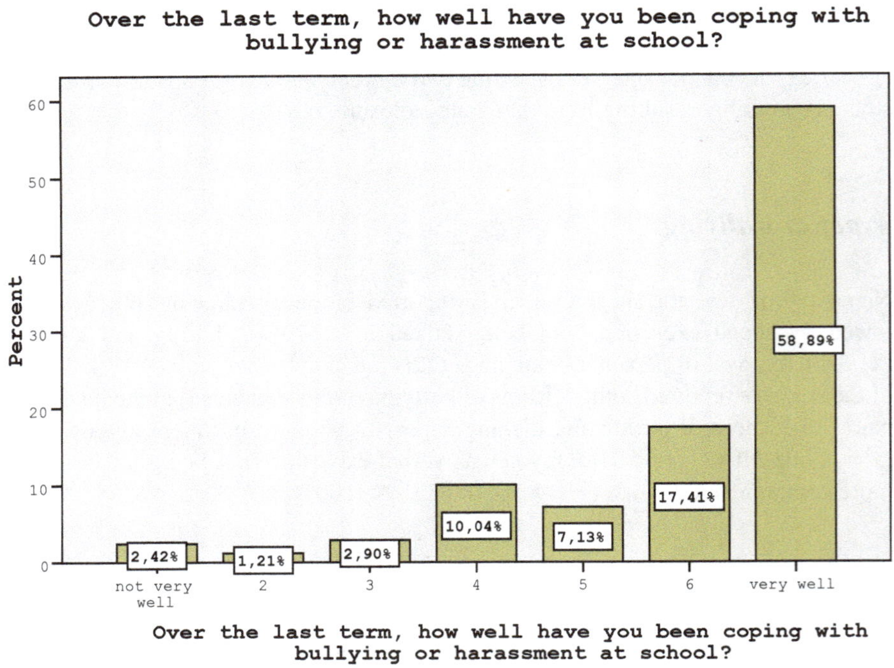

Fig. 6.1 Distribution of responses by participants on the self-efficacy scale

Neither gender nor mother language differences were found to exercise an effect on the reported self-efficacy of students; though older students reported slightly lower self-efficacy in coping with bullying (Spearman's rho = 0.12, $p < 0.001$, 2-tailed) when compared to their younger schoolmates.

Evaluating the Outcomes of the Anti-Bullying Program

The nonparametric Mann-Whitney *U* index revealed that the two groups of students (control and intervention groups) were not similar in terms of their initial rates of victimization ($U = 58{,}332$, N1 = 219, N2 = 630, $p < 0.001$, 2-tailed), with the intervention group reporting a higher rate of victimization. For this reason, a decision was made to exclude the control group from further analysis.

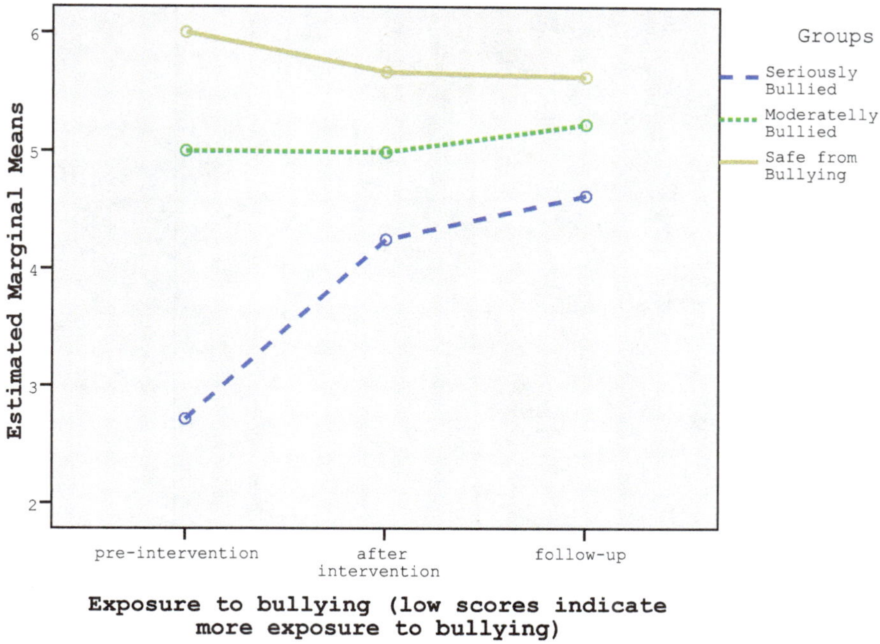

Fig. 6.2 The level of exposure to victimization of participants prior to intervention, post intervention, and upon follow-up

Exposure to Bullying, Perceived Safety, and Coping Efficacy

Exposure to Bullying

It was found that the timescale involved had a significant effect of on the level of exposure to victimization, $F(2, 968) = 47.25$, $p < 0.0005$, $\eta 2 = 0.089$). $F(2, 968) = 47.25$, $p < 0.0005$, $\eta^2 = 0.089$). There was also a significant interaction between the level of exposure students had to victimization in all repetitive measurements and in their initial rates of victimization $F(4, 968) = 59.52$, $p < 0.0005$, $\eta^2 = 0.197$). As shown in Fig. 6.2, the participants that were seriously bullied were transferred to safer zones and were most likely the ones who benefited most from intervention.

Perceived Sense of Safety from Being Bullied

By the end of the program, there was a significant increase in the reported sense of safety student felt, especially among those students who were seriously victimized. There was a slightly significant effect of time span on the students' perceived sense

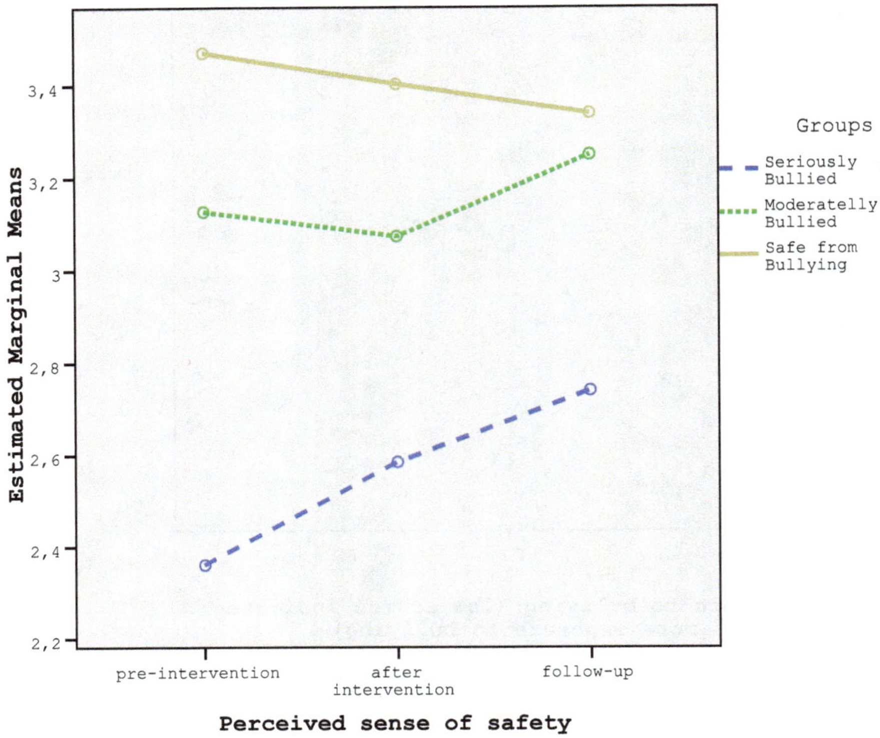

Fig. 6.3 The perceived sense of safety participants had prior to intervention, post intervention, and upon follow-up

of safety form being bullied $F(2, 964) = 2.65$, $p = 0.05$, $\eta^2 = 0.005$). Additionally, there was a significant correlation between the students' perceived sense of safety from being bullied across time and their initial extent of victimization $F(4, 964) = 4.48$, $p = 0.001$, $\eta2 = 0.018$). As shown in Fig. 6.3, at the end of the intervention, the seriously and moderately victimized students reported a greater sense of safety from being bullied.

Self-Efficacy in Coping with Bullying

Our next analysis concerned the outcomes reported by students and the intervention had on self-efficacy to counteract bullying. A significant interaction was found between the reported self-efficacy in tackling bullying over time and their initial rates of victimization $F(4, 910) = 4.89$, $p = 0.001$, $\eta2 = 0.021$). By the end of the program, students reported a significant increase in perceived effectiveness in combating victimization, especially among those children who were seriously and moderately bullied (see Fig. 6.4).

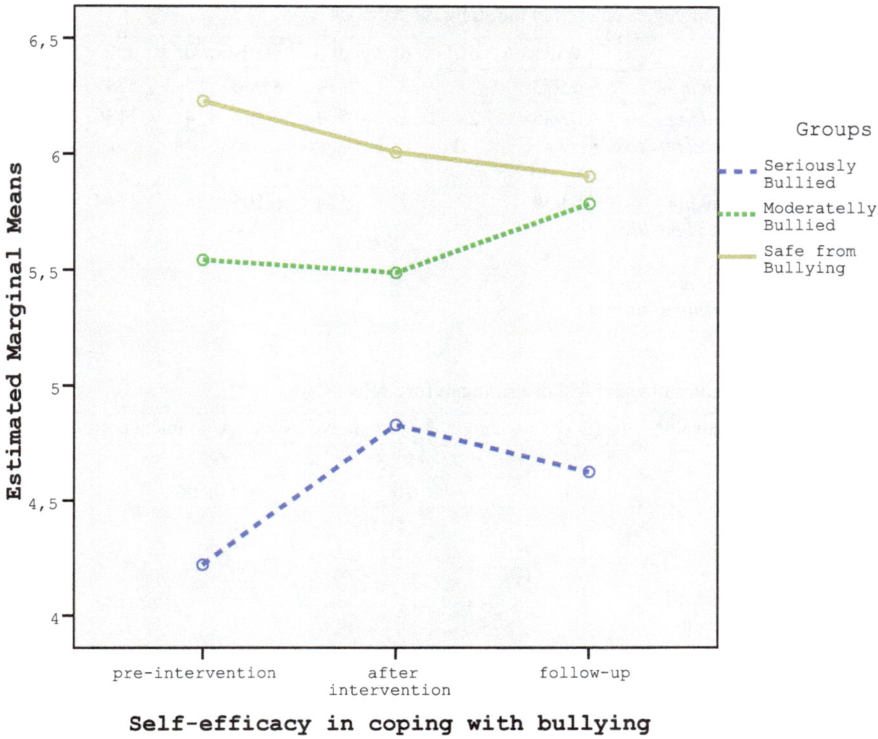

Fig. 6.4 The perceived efficacy of participants in coping with bullying prior to intervention, post intervention, and upon follow-up

Coping with Bullying

In order to determine how the various groups of students differed in terms of rates of victimization with regard to the coping strategies employed, we computed a discriminant function analysis, a stepwise method, which revealed two discriminant functions. The first explained 82.3% of the variance, canonical $R^2 = 0.224$, whereas the second explained only 17.7%, canonical $R^2 = 0.106$ (see Tables 6.4 and 6.5).

In combination, these two significant functions significantly differentiate between the treatment groups, $\Lambda = 0.939$, $\chi^2(6) = 36.117$, $p < 0.0005$. Whereas by removing the first function, the second function still significantly discriminates the treatment groups $\Lambda = 0.989$, $\chi^2(2) = 6.492$, $p < 0.05$. The correlations between the outcomes and discriminant functions revealed that the coping strategies of optimism and positive attitude loaded on both functions, fairly highly in the opposite direction on the first function ($r = -0.52$) and highly on the second function (r = 0.89). The strategies of *wishful thinking* and *pretending as if it is not happening* loaded highly

Table 6.4 Coping strategies entered in the stepwise statistics

Steps	Coping	Wilks' Λ	df 1	df 2	df 3	Statistic	df 1	df 2	Sig.
1	*Wishful thinking*	0.973	1	2	574	8.066	2	574	<0.0005
2	*Wishful thinking* *Optimism and positive attitude*	0.956	2	2	574	6.593	4	1146	<0.0005
3	*Wishful thinking* *Optimism and positive attitude* *Pretend as if not happening/submission*	0.939	3	2	574	6.105	6	1144	<0.0005

Table 6.5 Eigenvalues of canonical discriminant functions

Function	Eigenvalues	(%) of Variance	Cumulative (%)	Canonical correlation
1	0.05	82.3	82.3	0.224
2	0.01	17.1	100	0.106

Table 6.6 Standardized canonical discriminant function coefficients

	Function	
	1	2
Optimism and positive attitude	−0.525	0.894
Wishful thinking	0.731	0.165
Pretend as if not happening/submission	0.597	0.190

Table 6.7 Functions at group centroids

	Function	
Exposure to bullying level	1	2
Seriously bullied	0.662	−0.043
Moderately bullied	−0.024	0.182
Safe from bullying	−0.100	−0.065

on the first function ($r = 0.73$ and $r = 0.60$, respectively) and very low on the second function ($r = 0.73$ and $r = 0.60$, respectively) (Table 6.6).

According to the functions at group centroids shown in Table 6.7 and discriminant function plot (see Fig. 6.5), variate 1 discriminates the seriously bullied children from the other two groups (the moderately bullied and the safe group), and variate 2 discriminates the moderately bullied students from the remaining categories. Stated more simply, the seriously bullied students appear to adopt a less positive attitude toward handling bullying and rely more on the coping strategies of wishful thinking and pretending as if it is not happening. What seems to distinguish the moderately bullied students from their peers in other categories of victimization is the adoption of a more positive attitude (trying to be optimistic) in handling bullying.

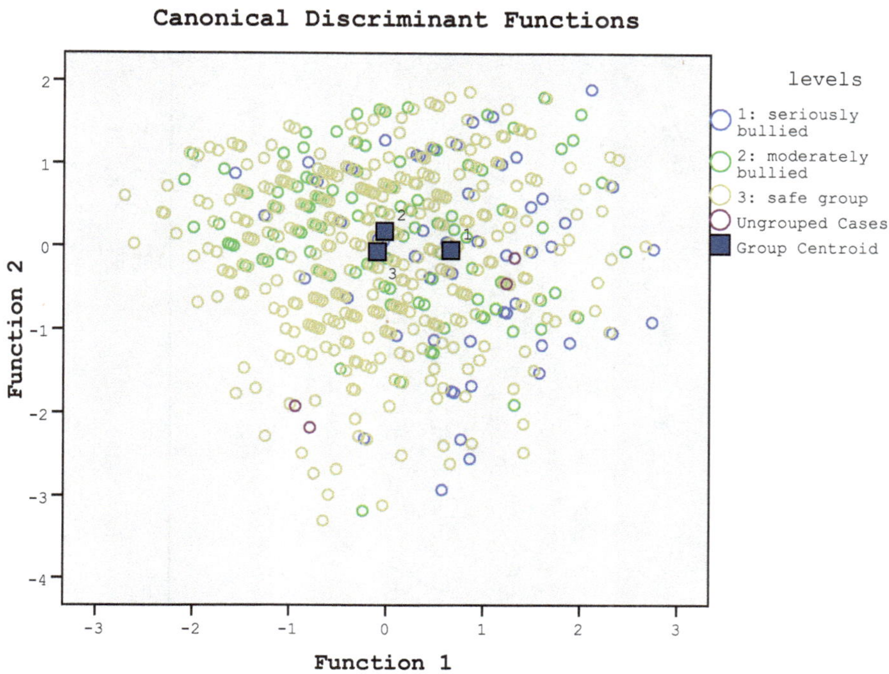

Fig. 6.5 Discriminant function plot of the rates of victimization among participants according to the coping strategies they use

Coping Strategies Before and After Intervention

From our results, it was found that three coping strategies are more closely linked to exposure to bullying including the expression of wishful thinking, pretending as if it is not happening/submission, and maintaining a positive attitude/optimism. Given that we found a significant decrease in exposure to bullying in the follow-up measurements, the mixed ANOVA design analysis that was conducted included only the coping strategies that were strongly correlated with high rates of victimization (as revealed by the discriminant function analysis).

Optimism and Positive Attitude Toward Bullying

The findings indicate that the main effect of time span on the frequency of use of the coping strategy of trying to be optimistic was significant, $F(2, 960) = 8.99$, $\eta 2 = 0.018$ $p < 0.0005$). There was no significant interaction between the coping strategy of happy try across time and the initial rates of student victimization $F(4, 960) = 0.47$, $p > 0.05$). As shown in Fig. 6.6, the three groups of students reported a reduction in the use of this particular coping strategy in similar ways.

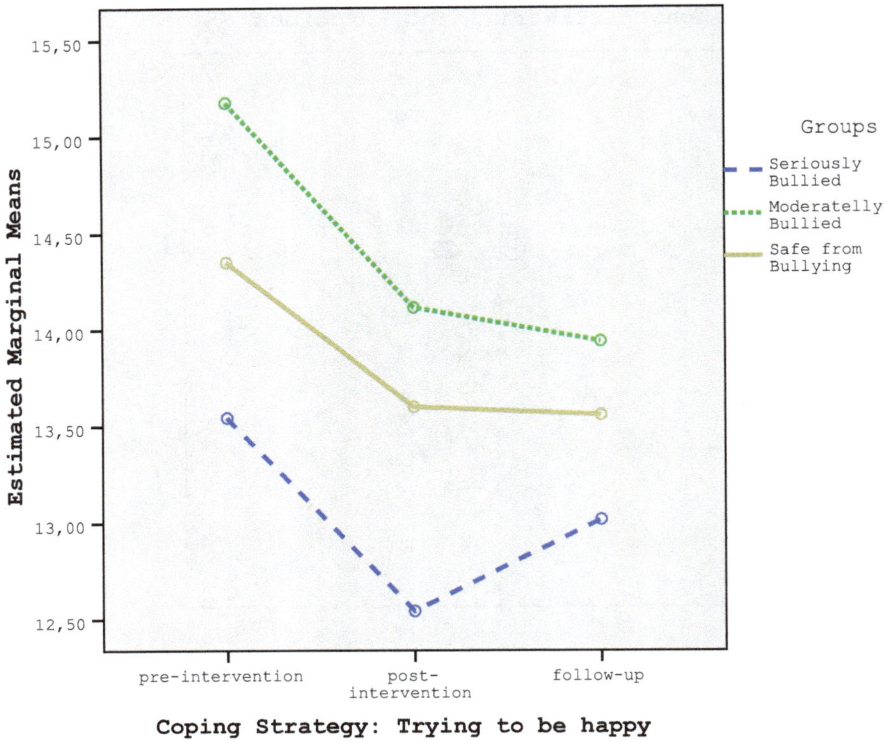

Fig. 6.6 Frequency of use by the participants of the coping strategies of being optimistic and maintaining a positive attitude, prior to intervention, post intervention, and upon follow-up

Wishful Thinking

A significant main effect of time on the frequency of use of the wishful thinking coping strategy was noted, $F(2, 952) = 18.77$, $\eta 2 = 0.04$, $p < 0.05$. No significant interaction of the coping strategy of wishful thinking across time and initial rates of students victimization was noted, $F(4, 952) = 0.53$, $p > 0.05$. As shown in Fig. 6.7, there was a reduction in the frequency of use of the wishful thinking coping strategy by all participants.

Pretend as if It Is Not Happening

There was evidence across repetitive measurements of a somewhat slightly significant main effect of time on the frequency of use of the strategy of pretending as if it is not happening, $F(2, 938) = 2.66$, $\eta^2 = 0.006$, $p = 0.05$. No significant interaction between the use of the coping strategy of pretending as if it is not happening

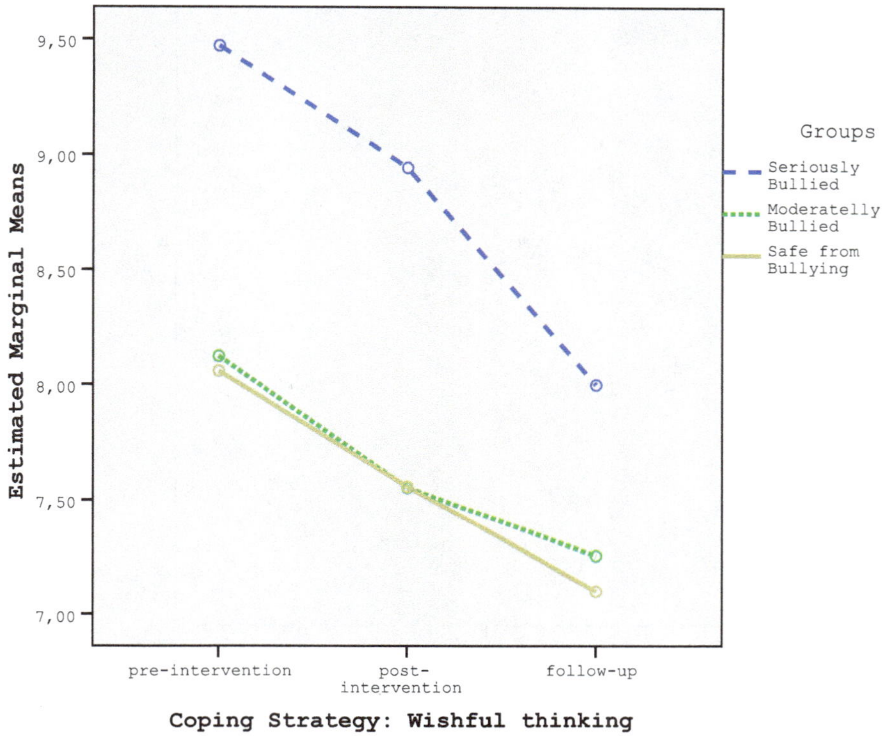

Fig. 6.7 Frequency of use by the participants of the coping strategy of wishful thinking prior to intervention, post intervention, and upon follow-up

across time and initial rates of students' victimization was found, $F(4, 938) = 0.51$, $p > 0.05$. Finally, as shown in Fig. 6.8, the frequency of use of the strategy of pretending as if it is not happening/submission was reduced in the case of all participants.

Discussion

The purpose of this research was to evaluate the effectiveness of the intervention program "coping with bullying at school" that was implemented in Greek high schools. The two main assumptions of our research were that: (a) the program would be effective, especially for the serious victimized students; and (b) the effects of the program on coping strategies would be particularly evident in tackling school bullying. Both of our main assumptions were not disputed. The program enhanced the students' sense of safety at their school, as well as their confidence in dealing with victimization. In particular, for those who reported serious victimization, the

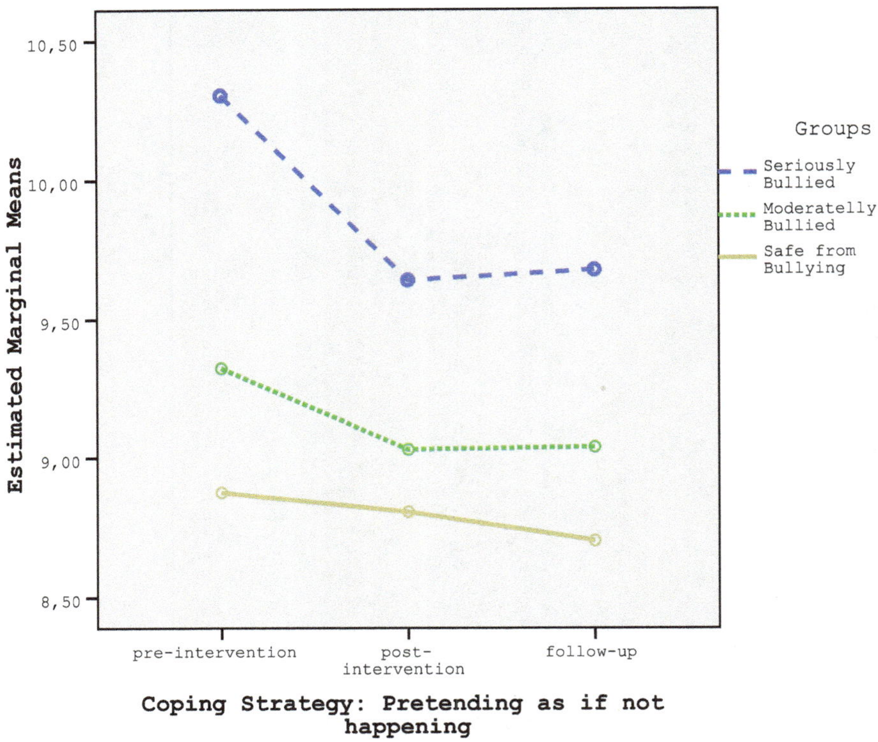

Fig. 6.8 Frequency of use by the participants of the coping strategy of pretending as if it is not happening/submission prior to intervention, post intervention, and upon follow-up

results showed that both at the end of the program and in repeated measurements, their exposure to victimization (based on their self-reporting) dropped significantly. There are many resonances between the outcomes of the program presented here and that reported in other contexts that implemented this particular intervention (Slee, 1996, 2005; Slee, Skrzypiec, & Murray-Harvey, 2009).

Seriously bullied children seem to engage more in wishful thinking, such as hope that the bullying will sort itself out or wish a miracle would happen. Serious exposure to bullying was also connected with a set of strategies including ignoring the bullies, pretend as it is not happening, avoid thinking about it, and give in to bullies. As pertinent evidence indicates systematically victimized students typically prefer and rely on counterproductive strategies for terminating their harassment by peers, such as crying, running away, or missing school (Paul, Smith, & Blumberg, 2012). Students who are seriously victimized seem to be less likely to applying problem-solving-oriented coping strategies that are highly recommended in many intervention programs, such as seeking help from an adult or peer or confronting the bullies in an assertive manner (Elledge et al., 2010; Skrzypiec, Slee, Murray-Harvey, &

Pereira, 2011; Terranova, 2009). Therefore, our findings in accordance with previous research evidence point to interventions that acknowledge the different needs of students within the school setting and question simplistic programs that underestimate the complex relation of bullying, coping, and well-being.

It's interesting that coping strategies such as seeking social support from an adult or peer and reacting emotionally toward other didn't prove to differentiate bullied from non-bullied children. This finding is in line with Bibou-Nakou and Markos (2013) but contrary to some other older studies (Houndoumadi & Pateraki, 2001; Hunter & Boyle, 2004) where classification was based on frequency measured either as a Likert scale measured from "everyday" to "never" or a measurement of the duration of bullying (e.g., more than 6 months). In addition, the data of the present study indicate there is no distinct set of strategies that can be effective for all types of victimization or likewise apply to all students. Most children and adolescents tend to rely on a combination of approaches for handling aggressive interactions with their schoolmates (Didaskalou et al., 2016; Murray-Harvey, Skrzypiec, & Slee, 2012; Tenenbaum, Varjas, Meyers, & Parris, 2011).

One of our striking findings is that what differentiates moderately bullied children from their seriously bullied peers is the use by the former of more "positive" coping strategies such as try to be cheerful despite the bullying, find ways to relax, think of different ways to solve the problem, and keep fit and healthy. Perhaps what makes the crucial difference between being seriously or moderately bullied is a depression-prone mental health profile. Although the correlation of prolonged exposure to bullying to mental health problems is well documented (e.g., Alikasifoglu, Erginoz, Ercan, Uysal, & Albayrak-Kaymak, 2007; Junoven & Graham, 2001), more research is needed in order to be established if the degrees of exposure to victimization reflect not only quantitative but also qualitative differences.

Regarding the changes observed in the strategies used by the seriously victimized group after the end of the intervention, there was an overall reduce in all three counterproductive coping with bullying strategies, for students of all three groups, although the effect sizes were quite low. Nevertheless, such a finding allows us to assume that any improvement of students' exposure to victimization might be associated with a reduction in the use of the abovementioned strategies that proved to be ineffective. However, the absence of control group in our study dictates special caution to be exercised when moving to any conclusion, as we cannot control time variables and other natural or due to maturation processes that are likely to affect the use of these strategies by students along with their exposure to risk for victimization.

Nevertheless, we can certainly argue that the structure, content, and materials of the program that we implemented identify school bullying as a real problem for which "something has to be done." Accordingly, the participants became fully aware about the ineffectiveness of strategies like pretending that bullying never occurred, hoping that it will go away, evading the bullies, and imaging that the bullies did not actually exist.

Although the intervention program had a great appeal within schools, we keep the constraints as made by Merrell, Gueldner, Ross, and Isava (2008), according to which intervention programs are likely to have a greater effect on students' knowledge, beliefs, and perceptions than their real behavior. On the other hand, we would also like to support further Cross and Barnes' (2014) reservations regarding the possibility of missing valuable information on what is actually happening in schools, when evaluating anti-bullying programs by simply using strict quantitative measures and criteria.

Based on the findings of our research, some questions have been answered, but some new questions have arisen that might be of interest to future studies. It was found that according to students' self-reporting, their level of exposure to victimization was reduced. However, when relying exclusively on students' self-reporting, socially desirability factors cannot be totally excluded. The present evidence needs therefore to be further substantiated by complementary observational data and relevant reports from teachers and classmates.

Additionally, verbal and physical bullying was reported very frequently by the participating students, even by those who had not been victimized. These findings raise concerns about the dominant norms and cultures within peer groups and the level of tolerance of aggressive attitudes in Greek high schools.

The schools involved in this study were predominantly favorably predisposed to the implementation of the intervention. It might therefore be important to investigate the particular characteristics that these schools are likely to share and investigate whether these differ in the schools not willing to participate.

Finally, it would be of particular interest to repeat this research in specialty schools, such as music and arts secondary schools, where artistic expression is integrated into peer relationships and interactions in a way that could serve as a regulatory or intermediate variable against victimization.

References

Alikasifoglu, M., Erginoz, E., Ercan, O., Uysal, O., & Albayrak-Kaymak, D. (2007). Bullying behaviours and psychosocial health: Results from a cross-sectional survey among high school students in Istanbul, Turkey. *European Journal of Pediatrics, 166*(12), 1253–1260.

Andreou, E., Roussi-Vergou, C., Zafiropoulou, M., Didaskalou, E., Skrzypiec, G., & Slee, P. (2012). *Coping with Bullying: A pilot intervention study*. Paper presented at the 13th Biennial Conference of the European Association for Research on Adolescence, Isle of Spetses, Greece.

Bibou-Nakou, I., & Markos, A. (2013). Coping strategies of secondary school students experiencing bullying: Frequencies, type of bullying and psychosocial difficulties. In K. Dekker & M. Dijkstra (Eds.), *School bullying: Predictive factors, coping strategies and effects on mental health* (pp. 69–96). New York, NY: Nova Science Publishers.

Clark – Carter, D. (2004). *Quantitative psychological research: A student's handbook*. East Sussex, UK: Psychology Press.

Cross, D., & Barnes, A. (2014). One size doesn't fit all: Re-thinking implementation research for bullying prevention. In R. M. Schott & D. M. Søndergaard (Eds.), *School bullying: New theories in context* (pp. 405–439). Cambridge, UK: Cambridge University Press.

Didaskalou, E., Roussi-Vergou, C., & Andreou, E. (2015). Greek adolescents' victimization experiences, reactions, ability to cope and sense of school safety. *American Journal of Psychology and Behavioral Sciences, 2*(2), 41–51.

Didaskalou, E., Skrzypiec, G., Andreou, E., & Slee, P. (2016). Taking action against victimization: Australian middle school students' experiences. *Journal of Psychologists and Counselors in schools, 27*(1), 106–122.

Elledge, L. C., Cavell, T. A., Ogle, N. T., Malcolm, K. T., Newgent, R. A., & Faith, M. A. (2010). History of peer victimization and Children's response to school bullying. *School Psychology Quarterly, 25*(2), 129–141.

Frydenberg, E., Lewis, R., Bugalski, K., Cotta, A., McCarthy, C., Luscombe-Smith, N., & Poole, C. (2004). Prevention is better than cure: Coping skills training for adolescents at school. *Educational Psychology in Practice, 20*(3), 117–134.

Houndoumadi, A., & Pateraki, L. (2001). Bullies and bullying in Greek elementary schools: Pupils' attitudes and teachers'/parents' awareness. *Educational Review, 53*(1), 19–26.

Hunter, S. C., & Boyle, J. M. (2004). Appraisal and coping strategy use in victims of school bullying. *British Journal of Educational Psychology, 74*, 83–107.

Junoven, J., & Graham, S. (2001). *Peer harassment at school: The plight of the vulnerable and the victimized*. New York, NY: Guilford Press.

Kanetsuna, T., Smith, P. K., & Morita, Y. (2006). Coping with bullying at school: Childrens recommended strategies and attitudes to school-based interventions in England and Japan. *Aggressive Behavior, 32*(6), 570–580.

Kochenderfer, B. J., & Ladd, G. W. (1997). Victimized children's responses to peers' aggression: Behaviors associated with reduced versus continued victimization. *Development and Psychopathology, 9*, 59–73.

Merrell, K. W., Gueldner, B. A., Ross, S. W., & Isava, D. M. (2008). How effective are school bullying intervention programs? A meta-analysis of intervention research. *School Psychology Quarterly, 23*(1), 26–42.

Murray-Harvey, R., Skrzypiec, G., & Slee, P. T. (2012). Effective and ineffective coping with bullying strategies as assessed by informed professionals and their use by victimised students. *Australian Journal of Guidance and Counselling, 22*(1), 122–138.

Murray-Harvey, R., & Slee, P. T. (2007). Supportive and stressful relationships with teachers, peers and family and their influence on students' social/emotional and academic experience of school. *Australian Journal of Guidance and Counselling, 17*(02), 126–147.

Newman, R. S. (2008). Adaptive and non adaptive help seeking with peer harassment: An integrative perspective of coping and self-regulation. *Educational Psychologist, 43*, 1–15.

Paul, S., Smith, P. K., & Blumberg, H. H. (2012). Comparing student perceptions of coping strategies and school interventions in managing bullying and cyberbullying incidents. *Pastoral Care in Education: An International Journal of Personal, Social and Emotional Development, 30*(2), 127–146.

Psalti, A. (2012). Bullies, victims and bully-victims in Greek schools: Research data and implications for practice. *Hellenic Journal of Psychology, 9*, 132–157.

Skrzypiec, G., Roussi-Vergou, C., & Andreou, E. (2011). Common problems, common solutions? Applying a foreign 'coping with bullying' intervention in Greek schools. In R. H. Shute, P. T. Slee, R. Murray- Harvey, & K. L. Dix (Eds.), *Mental health and wellbeing: Educational perspectives* (pp. 261–275). Adelaide, Australia: Shannon Research Press.

Skrzypiec, G., Slee, P., Murray-Harvey, R., & Pereira, B. (2011). School bullying by one or more ways: Does it matter and how do students cope? *School Psychology International, 32*(3), 288–311.

Skrzypiec, G., Slee, P., Roussi-Vergou, C., & Andreou, E. (2013). Coping with school bullying: A cross national pilot intervention study. *Journal of Modern Greek Studies, 3*, 232–245.

Slee, P. T. (2005). *The PEACE pack: Evaluation of a program for the successful reduction of school bullying. School bullying around the world*. Tokyo, Japan: Minerva Shobo Publishers.

Slee, P. T., Skrzypiec, G. K., & Murray-Harvey, R. (2009). *The coping with bullying intervention*. Paper presented at the ISSBD, Zambia.

Slee, R. (1996). Inclusive schooling in Australia? Not yet! *Cambridge Journal of Education, 26*(1), 19–32.

Smith, P. K., Talamelli, L., Cowie, H., Naylor, P., & Chauhan, P. (2004). Profiles of non-victims, escaped victims, continuing *victims and new victims of school bullying. British Journal of Educational Psychology, 74*(4), 565–581.
Tenenbaum, L. S., Varjas, K., Meyers, J., & Parris, L. (2011). Coping strategies and perceived effectiveness in fourth through eighth grade victims of bullying. *School Psychology International, 32*, 263–287.
Terranova, A. M. (2009). Factors that influence children's responses to peer victimization. *Child & Youth Care Forum, 38*, 253–271.
Van Deur, P. (2011). Seeking students' perspectives on their social and emotional wellbeing. In R. H. Shute, P. T. Slee, R. Murray- Harvey, & K. L. Dix (Eds.), *Mental health and wellbeing: Educational perspectives* (pp. 63–75). Adelaide, Australia: Shannon Research Press.

Chapter 7
Factors in Reporting Mobile Victimization in South African Schools

Michael Kyobe and Shallen Lusinga

Introduction

School-based violence and bullying are escalating today. Bullying is defined as "the exposure to negative actions which are done repeatedly and over time in a relationship where there is an imbalance of strength" (Olweus, 1997:497). Traditionally, the power imbalance is a key feature of bullying by which the aggressor tends to be physically, socially or psychologically more powerful than the victim (Orpinas & Horne, 2006). Cyberbullying refers to all forms of bullying committed using electronic means (Klomek, Sourande & Gould, 2010). In recent years, the proliferation of mobile phones has resulted in the escalation of mobile bullying, defined here as one form of cyberbullying committed using mobile technology (Livingstone, Stoilova & Kelly, 2016). The report by UNESCO and UN Women (2016) provides guidelines on how to deal with these challenges. One of the interventions is to encourage reporting bullying and other forms of aggression. Reporting violence and abuse in schools is particularly important in a country like South Africa, where the rate of crime is among the highest in the world (Cameron, 2016). However, victimization (by electronic means or otherwise) is under-reported, particularly in schools. This hampers efforts to combat anti-social behaviour (Pettalia et al., 2013; Styron, Bonner, Styron, Bridgeforth, & Martin, 2016). Understanding the factors contributing to failure to report bullying would contribute to the development of interventions that can reduce bullying and victimization (Styron et al., 2016). The objective of the present study is to examine the effects of various factors on reporting mobile victimization in South African schools. It also examines how the various

M. Kyobe (✉) · S. Lusinga
Department of Information Systems, University of Cape Town, Cape Town, South Africa
e-mail: michael.kyobe@uct.ac.za

J. U. Mofe Gordon (ed.), *Bullying Prevention and Intervention at School*,
https://doi.org/10.1007/978-3-319-95414-1_7

recommendations by UNESCO and UN Women (2016) on curbing SRGBV have been implemented by the South African government.

Literature Review

According to Goudriaan (2006), three theoretical models, namely, the economic, psychological and sociological models, have been used to investigate the determinants of reporting of crimes. Acknowledging the influence of technology on reporting of crimes, we also present the technological models. Each model focuses on a different mechanism and manifests at varying levels of Bronfenbrenner's (1979) ecological model, that is, the micro-, meso- and macro-level. These models are discussed further below.

Economic Model

The economic model assumes that people perform cost-benefit analyses before reporting a crime (Greenberg & Beach, 2004; Goudriaan, 2006). The victim determines whether reporting a crime is worth the effort. Victims would not, for instance, report crime when they perceive little action or help from law enforcement (Mtshazi & Kyobe, 2014). However, the economic model focuses more on the characteristics of the crime, such as the perceived seriousness of the crime, than on the social environment (Goudriaan, 2006). This model does not give consideration to the emotional and social processes which play a major role in the decision-making process of reporting crime (Greenberg & Beach, 2004).

Psychological Model

The psychological model posits that the decision to report crime is based on additional factors such as the social network of the victim (Goudriaan, 2006). The model claims that victims are too emotional or fearful to make rational decisions after a crime and as such "emotional arousal might influence victims' attention, perceptions, thoughts, judgments, and interpretations, processing capacity, and processing strategies" (Greenberg & Beach, 2004: 178). It has also been found that reporting a crime is affected by factors such as a victim's knowledge of the offender, as one may fear retribution by the offender (Goudriaan, 2006). Another important factor is the victim's social network, in that if a victim is advised to report by those to whom they are close, they are more inclined to do so.

While the psychological model focuses on the affective reactions of the victims and their social networks, it neglects the broader social contexts such as culture, which affects the networks of a victim (Ayodele & Aderinto, 2016). Researchers maintain that human decision-making and behaviour are influenced by the social and cultural contexts (Granovetter, 1985).

Sociological Model

The sociological model posits that the likelihood of reporting a crime is a function of the social structures that exist in the society in which the victim and offender live (Black, 1976). This model focuses on the contextual factors that influence reporting. Black (1976) argues that there are five social structural variables that influence reporting of victimization, from filing a complaint to legal officials up to the recognition of the victim. These social structural variables are stratification, morphology, culture, organization and social control (Black, 1976). Stratification refers to the uneven distribution of the conditions of existence such as food, access to land or water and money. Morphology refers to the distribution of people in relation to each other. Culture is the symbolic aspect relating to religion, decoration and folklore. Organization refers to the capacity for collective action, while social control refers to the response to deviant behaviour such as punishment, accusations, compensation and prohibitions.

In this paper, we focus more on the cultural influencers. Ayodele and Aderinto (2016) argue that consideration of cultural factors provides subjective explanations for reporting crime and may help in connecting victims to offenders and contextual situations. They maintain that in the African context, the individual household condition, communal values, attitudes and practices influence individual and communal safety and subsequently the reporting behaviour (Ayodele & Aderinto, 2016). UNESCO and UN Women (2016) also report that social and cultural norms such as fear of stigma, reprisal from partners and death tend to discourage reporting of SRGBV. Social and cultural norms can also influence the way teachers, school heads and policy-makers engage with students about gender, violence and sex issues (UNESCO & UN Women, 2016). Therefore, understanding cultural influences on reporting criminal behaviour is important in the development of intervention programmes (Rennison et al., 2011).

While the sociological model provides useful insight into the influence of social, structural and cultural factors, it ignores racial differences in criminal behaviours and generalizes effects across racial groups (Breetzke, 2010). Breetzke (2010) reports that racial differences in South Africa contribute to the high crime rates. The sociological model also neglects the individual decision-making process of reporting criminal behaviour and the direct and intermediate effects of the unique characteristics of a victim and their situation (Goudriaan, 2006). Walsh and Hemmens (2010) argue that while macro-level models are posited to investigate culture, they also tend to focus on group phenomenon, ignoring circumstances of individuals.

The focus of the present study is on factors influencing reporting bullying in a mobile communication environment. It is, therefore, appropriate to examine how technology contributes to under-reporting of cyber and mobile bullying.

Technological Models

Technology may either integrate into or interfere with everyday life (Swingle, 2016). Integration is when technology substitutes other methods due to its superior efficiency or improves an existing trait (Swingle, 2016). In the case of mobile technology, this can be facilitated through its ubiquity, context-sensitivity, identifying functions, and command and control functions. Pousttchi, Weizmann and Turowski (2003) explain how these features create value in their mobile added value (MAV) theory. Interference occurs when technology overrides an existing trait or overshadows a developmental phase (Swingle, 2016). Technology can interfere with psychosocial behaviours. It can accelerate negative or previously neutral behaviour to a point at which it becomes obsessive-compulsive (Swingle, 2016). Ndyave and Kyobe (2017) also show how mobile technology facilitates mobile bullying. The transformative nature of technology may be explained by the lifestyle and routine activities theory (LRAT). LRAT predicts that changes in legitimate opportunity structures, such as societally approved means to reach goals (Williams & McShane, 2010), can increase the convergence of motivated offenders and make young people suitable targets in the absence of capable guardianship (Pratt et al., 2010). Social networking technologies (SNTs) have become a commonly accepted means by which people communicate, do business, share ideas and develop themselves. However, the strong attachment to the technologies, the repeated access to the networks and the time spent on them continue to expose the youth to victimization (Marcum et al., 2010).

Lusinga and Kyobe (2017) used these dimensions to develop a typology that predicts victimization. This typology can be used to determine which victims are most likely to report or not. A victim is likely to report if he/she possesses an advanced mobile phone, is more attached to it and uses it more frequently. Victims' frequent use of phones has been identified as a predictor of likelihood to reporting victimization (Sidebottom, 2014). Cell phones have many features that facilitate reporting. They can also allow anonymous reporting, shorten the time to report, increase flexibility and lower reporting costs (Tolsma, Blaauw & Te Grotenhuis, 2012). Attachment to things has been associated with negative emotionality. Pauli-Pott, Haverkock, Pott and Beckmann (2007) found that in infants with high negative emotionality, there exists a stronger relationship between attachment disorganization and behaviour problems. A study by Ishii (2011) found that emotionality is significantly correlated with the frequency of mobile phone use and delinquency score; it is also associated with perceived addiction and the delinquent tendency. An earlier survey conducted in Japan by Tsushin involving nondelinquent and delinquent students revealed that delinquent students make more calls per day and send more emails than nondelinquent students (Samkange-Zeeb & Blettner, 2009). Also, studies have found that the chance of reporting is significantly impacted by negative emotionality (Posick, 2014).

Another example of how the transformative power of technology can be negative is shown in the use of SNTs. Neubaum (2016) found that the likelihood of reporting anti-social behaviour was strongly influenced by people's "fear of isolation". The fear of isolation draws attention to user-generated comments which result in their public opinion perceptions being affected. Neubaum (2016) also found that sanctions or attacks that people expect from others about expressing their opinions if they are in the minority affect a user's willingness to convey their opinions. In her Spiral of Silence theory, Elizabeth Noelle-Neumann (1974) explains this phenomenon as "… diminishing frequency of public opinion due to the fear of nonconformity with the opinion of the majority and the resulting prospects of isolation or sanctions" (Palekar et al., 2015: 4).

The discussion above indicates that the economic, psychological and sociological models for understanding crime reporting behaviours have strengths and fundamental shortcomings especially regarding their areas of emphasis and focus. These models have also been applied independently in previous studies. Bullying and factors contributing to the failure to report this aggression are complex and require a much broader model to guide their study. Also, the inclusion of technological models enhances understanding of reporting behaviour in a digital environment. It has been suggested that to understand human behaviour better, multifaceted approaches are necessary (Barker, 1968; Bursik & Grasmick, 1993). In South Africa, there remains significant under-reporting of electronic and traditional crime, including sexual offences and domestic violence (Mbalula, 2017). Sibanda-Moyo et al. (2017) argue, for instance, that victimization against women (VAW) in South Africa is still occurring in great numbers. Since 2002, South Africa has been ranked number one in the world with regard to reported cases of VAW (Sibanda-Moyo et al., 2017). These researchers call for multifaceted approaches that consider the socioeconomic realities of women (such as education, income and employment) and macro factors (such as patriarchal structures, social and economic policies that shape their lives and experiences), to address such aggression. They also call for the strengthening of the existing laws' implementation and accountability for those already in existence.

Towards an Integrative Theoretical Framework for Studying Factors Influencing Under-reporting

We begin the development of the integrative theoretical framework by considering Bronfenbrenner's (1979) socioecological model. This model serves as an overarching umbrella within which the complex factors and interactions that influence bullying behaviour can be examined and addressed (Pintado, 2006). The model considers the different individualistic, social, physical, institutional and community

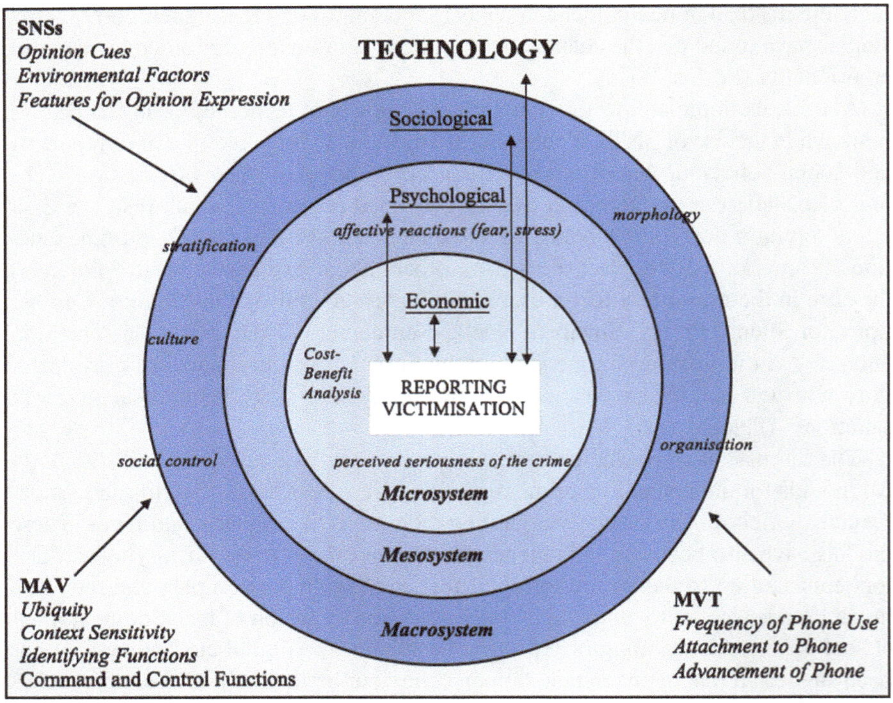

Fig. 7.1 Integrative framework for understanding reporting behaviour of mobile victims. (At each level of the integrative model, there are theories that help explain the victim's reporting behaviours. These include the four models presented above (i.e. economic, technological, social and psychological models): the lifestyle and routine activities theory (LRAT) and the MAV theory. MAV represents mobile added value (Pousttchi et al., 2003); SNSs represents attributes of social networking sites (Neubaum, 2016); and MVT represents dimensions of the mobile victimization typology (Lusinga & Kyobe, 2017)

aspects of bullying that affect young people (Pintado, 2006) and recognizes that youth exists in systems that directly, indirectly and dynamically affect their development (Lee, 2011). The ecological systems model consists of the microsystem, mesosystem and macrosystems. Microsystems involve interpersonal relationships that children may have (Lee, 2011). Mesosystems consist of social interconnections between participants, such as students, teachers and peers (Pintado, 2006). Macrosystems encompass the broad ideologies, attitudes, laws and customs of the culture that an individual falls in (Pintado, 2006).

Innumerable theories can be applied to the ecological systems framework—at different times, sequentially or simultaneously to assist understanding of why victims do not report victimization. Therefore, at each level of the ecological model, we identify theories that explain the victim's reporting behaviours. These behaviours may be explained by the economic, technological, social and psychological models, as well as the lifestyle and routine activities theory (LRAT) (Pratt et al., 2010). Taking these behaviours into consideration, the researchers have proposed the following integrative theoretical framework (Fig. 7.1) to guide the examination of the factors that influence reporting behaviour among victims of mobile bullying.

Methodology

As indicated earlier, a mobile application for monitoring and reporting mobile victimization was developed by the researchers and is currently being tested in schools. This application is based on the integrative theoretical model explained earlier and the victimization typology developed by Lusinga and Kyobe (2017). The application consists of information on victimization, a survey and reporting forms used by respondents to report victimization. This application is currently at the evaluation stage where we are establishing its effectiveness. One aspect of this evaluation, hence the aim of the present study, is to examine the effects of various factors on reporting mobile victimization in South African schools. The evaluation is conducted qualitatively using interviews with participating students. Qualitative research methods were considered more appropriate since they allow gathering more details about the participants and their social and cultural contexts within which they live (Myers, 1997). The target sample for this study was high school learners between the ages of 14 and 18 from both private and public schools in the Western Cape province of South Africa. The level of crime in this province is relatively high, and recent studies show that the use and abuse of mobile phones are escalating among South African youth (Creecy, 2012). Aftab (cited in Epstein & Kazmierczak, 2006) report that cyberbullying is prevalent in affluent suburbs. However, Oosterwyk (2013) also found the prevalence of mobile bullying to be high in schools located in crime-ridden areas. In these areas these are predominantly public schools. The present study was approved by both the University of Cape Town and the Western Cape Department of Education. High school principals from two different schools (School A, a public school, and School B, a private school) and learners' parents (guardians) then gave the researchers permission for learners to participate in the study as most of the learners in these schools were minors. Consent letters were sent to the schools, and 17 students participated in this study as they showed interest in being interviewed. To protect their identities, they are referred to as P#. Table 7.1 presents the demographic information of the students that were interviewed.

The data for the study were then collected using semi-structured interviews to maintain consistency of data collected from all participants as well as to give the interviewees the opportunity to elaborate or provide more relevant information if they choose to do so. The interviews lasted between 30 and 45 min each and were recorded (permission was granted by the research participants). These interviews were later transcribed by the researchers. The transcribed data was then coded and analysed using thematic analysis to identify concepts and themes linked to reporting

Table 7.1 Demographic information of students interviewed

School A					School B				
P	Gender	Grade	Age	Race	P	Gender	Grade	Age	Race
P1	Female	9	14 years-old	Coloured	P8	Female	8	13 years-old	Black
P2	Female	9	15 years-old	Coloured	P9	Female	9	14 years-old	Coloured
P3	Female	10	15 years-old	Black	P10	Male	9	15 years-old	Coloured
P4	Female	10	15 years-old	Coloured	P11	Female	10	15 years-old	Coloured
P5	Female	10	16 years-old	Black	P12	Male	10	15 years-old	Coloured
P6	Female	10	16 years-old	Black	P13	Male	10	16 years-old	White
P7	Female	11	17 years-old	Black	P14	Male	11	16 years-old	Coloured
					P15	Female	11	16 years-old	Coloured
					P16	Female	11	16 years-old	Coloured
					P17	Male	11	17 years-old	Coloured

and intervening mobile victimization. According to Braun and Clarke (2006: 79), "thematic analysis is a method for searching for, identifying, recording, analysing and reporting patterns (themes) within data" and therefore seemed appropriate for analysing the data collected.

Findings and Discussion

All the students interviewed had experienced some form of cyberbullying. This section will highlight findings from the thematic analysis on why students do not report their victimization, whom they report to should they choose to report and the digital means by which students report their victimization. The six phases of thematic analysis provided by Braun and Clarke (2006) were used to discover the themes to be discussed. This involved an iterative process through which the researchers familiarized themselves with the data through transcription, reading and rereading the data and making notes of initial ideas, generating initial codes by developing "labels" or codes to identify important features in the dataset, examining codes to identify broader patterns of meaning (themes) that were in line with the proposed integrated framework in Fig. 7.1 and reviewing identified themes (checking the themes against the coded extracts, dataset and the research objectives).

The following main and subthemes emerged from the dataset explaining why students do not report mobile victimization:

Theme (1), economic factors (pointless to report as there is no benefit in doing so; nothing changes or consequences for bullies are rarely severe enough).

Theme (2), psychological factors (fear; fear cuts across mediums; fear cuts across all racial groups; adults and schools do not take students seriously).

Theme (3), cultural and social factors (students do not involve adults right away; students prefer to figure it out themselves first, embarrassment, victim blaming).
Theme (4), technological factors (ineffective technological reporting tool, reports not acknowledged, poor response rate, anonymity).

These themes are discussed in the following sections.

Economic Factors

Nothing Changes/Consequences Are Rarely Severe Enough

The findings indicate that many of the students did not report bullying behaviours because they felt that it is pointless as there is no benefit in doing so (P3, P4, P6, P7, P8, P12, P16, P14). For example, P8 claimed that "… we don't want to say anything because we don't know what the point is of saying something when it can't exactly be fixed". P6 mentioned that the school had light punishment for bullying behaviour and she did not trust the school to deal with her victimization incident. P3, on the other hand, reported victimization to her mother and pointed out that reporting was not effective because in her experience, even after the bully was warned, the bully would only stop for a while but continue with his/her aggressive behaviours thereafter.

These findings indicate that there is a trade-off between reporting and not reporting, consistent with the economic model which predicts that the victim determines whether reporting a crime is worth it or not (Li, 2010).

Psychological Factors

Fear

Victims are too emotional or fearful to make rational decisions after a crime. Students did not report their victimization because they feared that the bullying will continue or will get worse once the accused bully realized he/she had been reported (P4, P9, P10, P13, P14, P15). P10 (coloured male) was concerned that if the bully got to know that "…you reported, could make it worse". P15 (coloured female) said "… the person may retaliate or do things … physically to me". Also, P13 (white male) said that even though reporting is anonymous, there could still be a fear of being attacked by the bully. The results also showed that the fear of a bully translated across mediums in that even when one was bullied online, further victimization could take place offline in reaction to reporting (P15, P4). P4 (coloured female) said, "… reporting someone that's bullying me online, ...that person can get you anywhere in school". P15 (coloured female) also stated that "… she [bully] would actually threaten to come to my school …".

It also appears that fear to report cuts across all the racial groups that participated in the study. This may be attributed to the general culture of fear that has gripped South Africa for years. According to SA News.gov.za (2011), violent crime in South Africa has roots in apartheid by which millions of boys and young men were exposed to humiliating police harassment and violent prison system (SA News.gov.za, 2011). During apartheid, the rule of law was also undermined by the state-sponsored violence in townships. These issues that are uniquely South African cultivated a culture of violence that has reproduced itself ever since (SA News.gov.za, 2011). This culture has led to distrust of authority figures and created fear and insecurity among the communities (Schonteich & Louw, 2001; SA News.gov.za, 2011).

Cultural and Social Factors

Another reason for not reporting victimization was that students did not want to involve adults (school staff and parents) in their matters (P8, P6, P4, P3). They showed a reliance on figuring things out on their own or among themselves. For example, P8 (black female) said that "if you don't feel strong enough to confront a person, you can talk to a friend … I don't like the idea of bringing in adults into that situation… you can just talk to that person (offender)". P4 (coloured female) and P3 (black female) said that reporting to a teacher is embarrassing. P6 (black female) said that "… telling them [teachers] about stuff that happened out of school … they [teachers] had nothing to do with them really". Only at times when there seems to be the severity of the bullying of a victim would students approach adults for assistance. P14 (coloured male) confirms this by saying "I wouldn't tell my parents … unless it's very bad …".

These responses came from black and coloured students who belong to a collectivist ethnic group. While lack of reporting crime among this ethnic group has been blamed on the perceived "unquestioning obedience" for elders, respect for elders among Africans is a cultural value with good intentions (Emeakaroha, 2002). The term "elder" represents parents, elderly relatives, neighbourhood elders, elders in the workplace and older adults in general. For many Africans, elders are believed to be the teachers and directors of the young. Emeakaroha (2002: 8) cites several Africans cultural beliefs as follows:

> Among the Efik, it is said: "The words of one's elders are greater than amulets", it means that they give more protection than the amulet does. … the Igbo say: He who listens to an elder is like one who consults an oracle. The oracles are believed to give the infallible truths. Thus the elders are also believed to say the truth, and their words and instructions are heeded to for the promotion of good behaviour among the young. … the elders are taken to be the repository of communal wisdom, … they have conceded leadership in the affairs of the people. One of the reasons for this is the nearness of the elders to the ancestors. And in the African concept, 'Legitimate power lay in the office sanctioned by ancestral norms, not in the person; and the person lost his right to exact obedience once he abused that office'.

Given the roles and responsibilities teachers and elders carry out in society, it is possible that some young people would find it rather embarrassing to approach the elders without having thought through the issues and their consequences.

Victim Blaming

We found instances where lack of reporting was attributed to victim blaming. In these cases, when these victims reported victimization, they too were disciplined, which discouraged further reporting (P1, P7, P17). For example, when P1 reported threats by a schoolmate over voice notes on WhatsApp, "Mr Peters said should anything like this happen again, he will have both of us suspended and make sure other schools don't accept us". This highlights that the victims also face consequences for their victimization. In case such as this, the bully may manipulate facts to get the victim in trouble as well. Most of these themes point to victim blaming, defined as "a devaluing act that occurs when the victim(s) of a crime or an accident is held responsible — in whole or in part — for the crimes that have been committed against them (CRCVC, 2009: 2). This blame can appear in the form of negative social responses from professionals, the media and immediate family members and other acquaintances (Bagshaw, Chung, Couch, Lilburn & Wadham, 2000). This has a negative impact on reporting victimization. However, technology can also be useful in providing evidence that the bully indeed committed the aggression (Law et al., 2012), and it can store information that can be shared.

Technological Factors

Technology Does Not Facilitate Efficient and Effective Means of Reporting

Most of the students felt that reporting digitally was ineffective. They find it insufficient when the action taken is to delete a bully's post, comment or account. P1 thought the digital reporting facilities were not effective "… because most people can just create new accounts … It's like they're not stopping them from doing it again". P16 also said that "you have the power to report that person but … after they are suspended, they can just come back and that's nothing".

Although many of the SNSs have implemented and continuously update their policies, guidelines and tools to aid in reporting bullying behaviour, most students do not use these when they are victimized even though many are aware of their existence, especially for Facebook, Instagram and Snapchat. However, two coloured female students indicated having used the tools and found them effective. P4, who had used the reporting facilities online, said: "Yes … recently when I went back on my old account, I saw something about 'your report has been acknowledged, and we have cleared the problem' ...". P9 also claimed that it was effective in that they closed the bully's account instantly. She said "… I reported it to a group of friends, so I think many people reported it, that's why it was so effective".

Students also felt that unless there were other people reporting as well, their reports were not taken into consideration. P16 and P3 also agree that the reporting tool would be more effective if more people reported. However, P6 felt that these applications are not effective as they do nothing after a report has been received. She said "… you report it and you don't get a reply … nobody gets to listen to me … so what's the point of me reporting …". When asked if getting a response would suffice to her reporting, she said "… obviously, every platform that you report to does that, but we want a result about what has been done about it. How has the situation been approached?". This also highlights the automatic responses that these applications have been found to send to users who report. There is definitely a lack of human interaction; students want to be heard, and auto responses to reporting do not seem to do so.

The comments by P3, P6, P9 and P16 suggest that victims would rather not report digitally as their opinions would be insignificant. This resonates with the spiral of silence theory, i.e. if one's opinion is in the minority, it is silenced. Therefore, reporting using technology may encourage silence regarding victimization or abuse if victimization is experienced and reported by one individual. Another challenge to reporting is that technology makes the bully anonymous (P7, P9 and P17).

Who do students report to when they are cyber or mobile victimized?

Students mainly report their victimization to their friends, parents or staff at the school as explained below.

Reporting to Friends

Only two students reported victimization to their friends. For example, P15 said "yeah so now I can tell someone especially like my boyfriend because we are kind of very close … I would tell him…". Our findings are consistent with those of Patchin and Hinduja (2006) and Slonje and Smith (2008).

Reporting to Parents

Some students reported their victimization to their parents (P5, P9, P14, P15). For example, P5 said after telling her mother, "she said 'don't let it get you down, don't let it bother you because you don't know the person so you can't feel like you did anything wrong…".

Reporting to the School

Some students report their victimization to the schools (P1, P3, P4, P5). Students also indicated that in more serious cases, the schools take the issue to bully's parents. For example, P4 said "they [school officials] go confront the parents".

In some cases, regardless of race, many students resorted to blocking their bullies, ignoring them and forgetting about it, especially on WhatsApp (P2, P4, P5, P8, P10, P12, P13). For example, P10 indicated that blocking the bully and forgetting about the incident were best options.

How South Africa Has Responded to SRGBV Recommendations.

Since the status of children has been raised to the legal status of right holders, the government is now accountable as the principal duty bearer, and children's well-being has become a high priority for the South African government (Savahl et al., 2015). The Department of Basic Education (DBE) has thus signed a protocol with the South African Police Service (SAPS), whereby schools with violence and safety issues are linked to the SAPS, and the school principals may obtain an immediate response from the police when an incident is reported. Schools from six provinces have been linked to SAPS, and linking the remaining schools in the other provinces is underway (Parliamentary Monitoring Group, 2017). Also, the DBE has drafted policies on use of alcohol and guidelines for drug testing and doping which have been submitted to UNICEF for final inputs before they could be implemented (Parliamentary Monitoring Group, 2016).

These efforts build on the already established legal commitments which include South Africa's ratification of the United Nations Convention on the Rights of the Child (UNCRC) and the establishment of the National Programme of Action for Children (NPAC) by the Office of the Rights of the Child (ORC). Also, the legal commitments to protect children's rights are already in place such as the Development of the Children's Act (2005), the Children's Amendment Act (2007) and the Child Justice Act (2008); all these commitments demonstrate South Africa's leadership role in protecting children's right (Savahl et al., 2015).

There are, however, still disparities that exist within children of differing socioeconomic status (SES) groups. Children in low-SES groups in particular still face high exposure to violence and domestic abuse, poor educational outcomes, health care and other services. The invasion of gangs into schools, bullying and abuse of teachers also raise concerns. The overall public safety in South Africa also compounds some of these issues as the children live in environments characterized by low public safety. Statistics released in 2017 indicate that for the sixth consecutive year, there has been an increase in robbery and murder incidents (Lancaster, 2017). While the government of South Africa has provided more resources to the police force, many challenges in the fight against crime and abuse persist. It is complicated even more by the fact that victims of crime are not reporting to the police (Lancaster, 2017).

The DBE in collaboration with UNICEF has been working on developing child-friendly school programmes (Parliamentary Monitoring Group, 2015).

Unfortunately, this endeavour has faced challenges with regard to physical infrastructure and equipment, safety and security, management and governance and partnerships. The DBE has also worked with the Centre for Justice and Crime Prevention (CJCP) to create and roll out early warning systems and guide and management tool for principals, school management teams and school governing bodies.

At the school level, the DBE is working with its legal services to ensure mandatory implementation of the National Safe Schools Framework (NSSF) by schools. Schools are also compelled to do a safety risk assessment twice a year. Also, every school would need to have an emergency plan and a disaster management plan and ensure that learners are supervised throughout the school day and after school hours, especially when schools go on excursions. To assist with cyberbullying, with support from Microsoft South Africa and Intel, the DBE developed and circulated a manual on cyberbullying for and in schools. The DBE also conducted an institutional and systemic programme to address bullying in schools which included trainers, who in turn trained teachers on how to deal with bullying. Training manuals have been developed and distributed in schools to support this strategy (Parliamentary Monitoring Group, 2017). To ensure learners are not left out, the school curriculum has been revised to include anti-bullying lessons, among others, as part of the life orientation subject (eNCA.com, 2017). Currently, the DBE is working together with many social partners to develop a "behaviour change" communications campaign, in order to communicate key messages to the public.

Conclusion

This study examined the factors influencing mobile victimization reporting by high school students in South Africa. Reporting crime is considered one effective way of combating cyberbullying and victimization. The preliminary findings of the present study confirm the complexity of the factors influencing students decision to (or not to) report aggression. Students do not report their victimization because of economic, psychological, cultural-sociological and technological factors, as predicted by our integrative theoretical framework. This implies, therefore, that our integrative theoretical framework is not only valuable in explaining the broad social-cultural context of victimization reporting but also in reporting behaviours at the individual level. The framework can, therefore, be used to guide further examination of the problem of under-reporting cyber victimization and inform the development of appropriate interventions in schools and communities.

Cultural and social factors, however, appear to be the most common influencers of victimization reporting in South African schools. The study revealed that students prefer to resolve issues themselves and only report to adults when they fail. This contradicted the earlier claim that ethnical demands on young Africans, such as unquestioning obedience and respect for elders and teachers, make them fail to disclose victimization for fear of being perceived to be disrespectful. African cultural practices are, however, intended to prepare the youth for responsible roles and to condition them to deal with challenges with limited intervention by elders (Emeakaroha, 2002; Olawoye et al., 2004). Obedience to the elders by the youth is not necessarily based on fear but on the fact that they (the youth) consider the elders to be custodians of wisdom, their social guides, teachers, promoter of good behaviour and judges (Olawoye et al., 2004). It, therefore, follows that the youth would find it appropriate to think through the issues first before engaging or reporting to the elders.

We are concerned that students found reporting victimization using digital means ineffective. While we agree that mobile technology has limitations, there is evidence that the interference of technology in the criminal justice system has been beneficial, especially at the reporting stage. Technologies, particularly mobile technologies, provide stored depictions and evidence to support reports of crime and encourage law enforcement to pursue cases (Boux & Daum, 2015). Earlier researchers concur that interventions in the form of new technical developments can make a difference in intervening bullying (Slonje, Smith & Frisén, 2013). We must emphasise, though, that for mobile technology and social media to be beneficial, effective interactions between the victims and the technology, service providers and other actors (like teachers) are critical. Automatic responses generated by mobile applications are not that helpful.

We commend the South African government and the DBE for the interventions put in place to address SRGBV recommendations. However, there are still major persistent challenges such as high exposure to violence and domestic abuse, poor educational outcomes and others revealed in the 2017 Police crime report (Mbalula, 2017). These create fear among the youth and consequently prevent victimization reporting. More effective strategies are needed to address these issues. For instance, while the DBE is playing a powerful role in schools and school communities, Styron et al. (2016) argue that parental or guardian involvement may lead to effective interventions. Our findings showed that only when there is severity in the bullying incidences do students report to adults, especially their parents. We, therefore, encourage the parents and guardians of students to be involved in the efforts of the DBE, not only when the consequences of bullying are severe but throughout the bullying experiences their children may be facing. Also, since not many digital tools have been developed to address the mobile victimization problem in South Africa, we encourage the development of interventions in the form of new technologies to fit the uniquely South African context whose past in apartheid strongly influences how people deal with processes in the legal or justice system (Schonteich & Louw, 2001; SA News.gov.za, 2011).These developments must, therefore, consider and cater to the different cultural contexts in South Africa and to its past in order for them to be useful, effective and efficient.

This study is not without limitations. The findings presented are preliminary and are based on the newly developed theoretical framework. This study also analysed data from a sample that had greater numbers of one collectivist ethnic group than others. Future studies should, therefore, test the framework using a large-scale study across schools from various safety zones. Doing so would ensure greater insight into the factors that influence victimization reporting, especially the cultural influences on reporting of different types of ethnic groups in South Africa. This would also further develop and establish the proposed integrative framework theoretically and confirm its contributions to the studies of mobile victimization reporting.

References

Ayodele, J. O., & Aderinto, A. A. (2016). Socio-cultural conditions of victims and their crime reporting practices in Lagos, Nigeria. *African Journal of Criminology and Justice Studies: AJCJS, 9*(1), 207–242.

Bagshaw, D., Chung, D., Couch, M., Lilburn, S., & Wadham, B. (2000). *Reshaping responses to domestic violence*. Adelaide, Australia: University of South Australia.

Barker, R. G. (1968). *Ecological psychology: Concepts methods for studying the environment of human behavior*. Stanford, CA: Stanford University Press.

Black, D. J. (1976). *The behavior of law*. New York, NY: Academic Press.

Boux, H. J., & Daum, C. W. (2015). At the intersection of social media and rape culture: How Facebook postings, texting and other personal communications challenge the real rape myth in the criminal justice system. *Journal of Law, Technology, and Policy, 1*(2015), 149–186.

Braun, V., & Clarke, V. (2006). Using thematic analysis in psychology. *Qualitative Research in Psychology, 3*(2), 77–101.

Breetzke, G. (2010). A socio-structural analysis of crime in the city of Tshwane, South Africa. *South African Journal of Science, 106*(11–12), 1–7.

Bronfenbrenner, U. (1979). *The ecology of human development*. Cambridge: Harvard university press.

Bursik, R. J. & Grasmick H. (1993). *Neighborhoods and crime: The dimensions of effective community control*. Lexinton, MA: Lexington Books.

Cameron, J. (2016). *South Africa's shock crime statistics: More worrying than corruption? Expert analysis*. Retrieved from http://www.biznews.com/leadership/2016/09/13/south-africas-shock-crime-statistics-more-worrying-than-corruption-expert-analysis/

CRCVC. (2009). *Victim Blaming*. Retrieved from http://crcvc.ca/docs/victim_blaming.pdf

Creecy, B. (2012). *Gauteng education MEC Barbara Creecy's opening address at the colloquium on bullying at Turffontein Racecourse 21 August 2012*. Retrieved from http://www.education.gpg.gov.za/Media/Statements/Documents/Media%20Statement%20-%20MEC%20address%20at%20colloquium%2021%20August%202012.pdf

Emeakaroha, E. (2002). *Seminar Paper presented by Rev. Fr. Dr. Emeka Emeakaroha On the 14th of* March 2002 *At the Theological department of the University of Vienna Austria*. Retrieved from http://www.emeka.at/african_cultural_vaules.pdf

eNCA.com. (2017). *Reports of bullying in Gauteng schools on the rise*. Retrieved from https://www.enca.com/south-africa/reports-bullying-gauteng-schools-rise

Epstein, A., & Kazmierczak, J. (2006). Cyberbullying: What teachers, social workers, and administrators should know. *Illinois child welfare, 3*(1– 2), 41–51.

Goudriaan, H. (2006). *Reporting crime: Effects of social context on the decision of victims to notify the police*. Heike Goudriaan.

Granovetter, M. (1985). Economic action and social structure: The problem of embeddedness. *American Journal of Sociology, 91*(3), 481–510.

Greenberg, M. S., & Beach, S. R. (2004). Property crime victims' decision to notify the police: Social, cognitive, and affective determinants. *Law and Human Behaviour, 28*(2), 177–186.

Ishii, K. (2011). Examining the adverse effects of mobile phone use among Japanese adolescents. *Keio Communication Review, 33*(2011), 69–83.

Klomek, A. B., Sourander, A., & Gould, M. (2010). The association of suicide and bullying in childhood to young adulthood: A review of cross-sectional and longitudinal research findings. *The Canadian Journal of Psychiatry, 55*(5), 282–288.

Lancaster, L. (2017). *Why are South Africans underreporting on crime?* Retrieved from https://issafrica.org/iss-today/why-are-south-africans-underreporting-on-crime

Law, D., Shapka, J., Hymel, S., Olson, B., & Waterhouse, T. (2012). The changing face of bullying: An empirical comparison between traditional and internet bullying and victimization. *Computers in Human Behavior, 28*(1), 226–232.

Lee, C. H. (2011). An ecological systems approach to bullying behaviors among middle school students in the United States. *Journal of Interpersonal Violence, 26*(8), 1664–1693.

Li, Q. (2010). Cyberbullying in high schools: A study of students' behaviors and beliefs about this new phenomenon. *Journal of Aggression, Maltreatment & Trauma, 19*(4), 372–392.

Livingstone, S., Stoilova, M., & Kelly, A. (2016). Cyberbullying: Incidence, trends and consequences. In *Ending the torment: Tackling bullying from the Schoolyard to Cyberspace* (pp. 115–120). New York, NY: United Nations Office of the Special Representative of the Secretary-General on Violence against Children.

Lusinga, S., & Kyobe, M. (2017). Testing a typology of mobile phone victimisation using cluster analysis. *The Electronic Journal of Information Systems in Developing Countries, 78*(6), 1–36.

Marcum, C., Higgins, G., & Ricketts, M. (2010). Potential factors of online victimization of youth: An examination of adolescent online behaviours utilizing routine activity theory. *Deviant Behavior, 31*(5), 381–410.

Mbalula, F. (2017). *Minister Fikile Mbalula – Speech at the Gender-Based Violence And Protection of Vulnerable Groups*. Retrieved from http://www.policesecretariat.gov.za/newsroom/speeches/MINISTER_FIKILE_MBALULA_SPEECH_AT_THE_GENDER_BASED_VIOLENCE_AND_PROTECTION_OF_VULNERABLE_GROUPS.pdf

Mtshazi, S., & Kyobe, M. (2014). *Investigating the role of the law enforcement in combating mobile bullying in South African high schools*. Retrieved from http://www.ictforafrica.org/images/stories/downloads/ICT4A2014Proceddings/ConferencePapers/ict4a-84-%20mtshazi.pdf .

Myers, M. D. (1997). Qualitative research in information systems. *Management Information Systems Quarterly, 21*(2), 241–242.

Ndyave, Z. C., & Kyobe, M. (2017). Factors that influence mobile bully-victim behaviour on social media: The case of Facebook. *Journal of Advances in Information Technology, 8*(4), 230–233.

Neubaum, G. (2016). *Monitoring and expressing opinions on social networking sites empirical investigations based on the spiral of silence theory.* Doctoral dissertation, University of Duisburg-Essen.

Noelle-Neumann, E. (1974). The spiral of silence a theory of public opinion. *Journal of Communication, 24*(2), 43–51.

Olawoye, J. E., Omololu, F. O., Aderinto, Y., Adeyefa, I., Adeyemo, D., & Osotimehin, B. (2004). Social construction of manhood in Nigeria: implications for male responsibility in reproductive health. *African population studies, 19*(2), 1–20.

Olweus, D. (1997). Bully/victim problems in school: Facts and intervention. *European Journal of Psychology of Education, 12*(4), 495–510

Oosterwyk, G. (2013). *Mobile bullying in South Africa – Exploring its nature, influencing factors and implications*. Masters Dissertation, University of Cape Town, Cape Town.

Orpinas, P., & Horne, A. (2006). *Bullying prevention: Creating a positive school climate and developing social competence*. Washington, D.C.: American Psychological Association.

Palekar, S., Atapattu, M., Sedera, D., & Lokuge, S. (2015). *Exploring spiral of silence in digital social networking spaces* (p. 2015). Fort Worth, TX: Thirty Sixth International Conference on Information Systems.

Parliamentary Monitoring Group. (2015). *School Safety/Violence & Bullying in Schools; Quality Learning and Teaching Campaign (QLTC) Implementation: progress report*. Retrieved from https://pmg.org.za/committee-meeting/21219/

Parliamentary Monitoring Group. (2016). *Department of Basic Education on its 2015/16 Annual Report, in presence of Minister & Deputy Minister*. Retrieved from https://pmg.org.za/committee-meeting/23528/

Parliamentary Monitoring Group. (2017). *Safety in Schools: DBE & SAPS briefing; Feedback on KZN Oversight Visit*. Retrieved from https://pmg.org.za/committee-meeting/25230/

Patchin, J. W., & Hinduja, S. (2006). Bullies move beyond the schoolyard: A preliminary look at cyberbullying. *Youth Violence and Juvenile Justice, 4*(2), 148–169.

Pauli-Pott, U., Haverkock, A., Pott, W., & Beckmann, D. (2007). Negative emotionality, attachment quality, and behavior problems in early childhood. *Infant Mental Health Journal, 28*(1), 39–53.

Pettalia, J. L., Levin, E., & Dickinson, J. (2013). Cyberbullying: Eliciting harm without consequence. *Computers in Human Behavior, 29*(6), 2758–2765.

Pintado, I. (2006). *Perceptions of school climate and bullying in middle schools*. Doctoral dissertation, University of South Florida.

Posick, C. (2014). Victimization and reporting to the police: The role of negative emotionality. *Psychology of violence, 4*(2), 210–223.

Pousttchi, K., Weizmann, M., & Turowski, K. (2003). *Added value-based approach to analyze electronic commerce and mobile commerce business models*. 2003 Proceedings International Conference Management and Technology in the New Enterprise, La Habana, Cuba. Del 22 al 25 de Abril del 2003, 414–423.

Pratt, T., Holtfreter, K., & Reisig, M. (2010). Routine online activity and internet fraud targeting: Extending the generality of routine activity theory. *Journal of Research in Crime and Delinquency, 47*(3), 267–296.

Rennison, C. M., Gover, A. R., Bosick, S. J., & Dodge, M. (2011). Reporting violent victimization to the police: A focus on Black, White, Asian, and Hispanic adolescent victims. *The open family studies journal, 4*(2011), 54–67.

Samkange-Zeeb, F., & Blettner, M. (2009). Emerging aspects of mobile phone use. *Emerging Health Threats Journal, 2*(1), 7082.

SA News.gov.za. (2011). *SA's violent crime has roots in apartheid, says report*. Retrieved from http://www.sanews.gov.za/features/sas-violent-crime-has-roots-apartheid-says-report

Savahl, S., Adams, S., Isaacs, S., Hendricks, G., Matzdorff, A., Wagenaar, C., Abrahams, L., & September, R. (2015). *Children's Worlds National Report: South Africa*. Children's Worlds Project. Retrieved from http://www.isciweb.org/_Uploads/dbsAttachedFiles/SouthAfrica_NationalReport_Final.pdf

Schonteich, M., & Louw, A. (2001). *Crime in South Africa: A country and cities profile*. Institute for Security Studies Papers: Pretoria, South Africa, 2001(49).

Sibanda-Moyo, N., Khonje, E., & Kyerewaa Brobbey, M. (2017). Violence against women in South Africa, A Country In Crisis. Retrieved from http://www.csvr.org.za/pdf/Full-report-to-client.pdf

Sidebottom, A. (2014). On the correlates of reporting assault to the police in Malawi. *British Journal of Criminology, 55*(2), 381–398.

Slonje, R., & Smith, P. K. (2008). Cyberbullying: Another main type of bullying? *Scandinavian Journal of Psychology, 49*(2), 147–154.

Slonje, R., Smith, P., & Frisén, A. (2013). The nature of cyberbullying, and strategies for prevention. *Computers in Human Behavior, 29*(1), 26–32.

Styron, R. A., Jr., Bonner, J. L., Styron, J. L., Bridgeforth, J., & Martin, C. (2016). Are teacher and principal candidates prepared to address student cyberbullying? *Journal of At-Risk Issues, 19*(1), 19–28.

Swingle, M. (2016). *i-Minds: How cell phones, computers, gaming, and social media are changing our brains, our behavior, and the evolution of our species*. Gabriola, Canada: New Society Publishers.

Tolsma, J., Blaauw, J., & Te Grotenhuis, M. (2012). When do people report crime to the police? Results from a factorial survey design in the Netherlands, 2010. *Journal of Experimental Criminology, 8*(2), 117–134.

UNESCO, & UN Women. (2016). *Global guidance on addressing school-related gender-based violence*. New York, NY: UNESCO Publishing.
Walsh, A., & Hemmens, C. (2010). *Introduction to criminology: A text/reader*. Thousand Oaks, CA: Sage.
Williams III, F. P., & McShane, M. D. (2010). *Criminology theory: Selected classic readings*. Cincinnati, OH: Anderson Publishing Co.

Chapter 8
Measuring Bullying Prevention and Intervention

Jacob U'Mofe Gordon

Problems of Definition

Evaluation is a systematic determination of a subject's merit, worth, and significance, using criteria governed by a set of standards. It can assist an organization, program, project, or any other intervention on initiative to assess any aim, realizable concept/proposal, or any alternative, to help in decision-making, or to ascertain the degree of accomplishment or value in regard to the aim and objectives and results of any such action that has been completed.

The primary purpose of evaluation, in addition to gaining insights into prior or existing initiatives, is to enable reflections and assist in the identification of future change. Evaluation looks at original objectives and at what is either predicted or what was accomplished and how it was accomplished; simply put, it helps to determine what works and why. Thus, evaluation can be formative, which is taking place during the development of concepts/proposals, project, or organization, with the intention of improving the value or effectiveness of the proposal, project, or organization. Evaluation can also be summative, that is, by drawing lessons from a completed or project or an organization at a later point in time or circumstances. Evaluation is inherently a theoretically informed approach (whether explicitly or not), and consequently any particular definition of evaluation must be tailored to its context—the theory, needs, purpose, and methodology of the evaluation process itself. Evaluation has also been defined by other scholars as:

> A systematic, rigorous, and meticulous application of scientific methods to assess the design, implementation, improvement, or outcomes of a program.

J. U. Gordon (✉)
University of Kansas, Lawrence, KS, USA

University of Ghana, Accra, Ghana

J. U. Gordon (ed.), *Bullying Prevention and Intervention at School*,
https://doi.org/10.1007/978-3-319-95414-1_8

Ross et al. (2004) remind us that evaluation is a resource-intensive process, frequently requiring resources, such as evaluation expertise, labor, time, and a sizable budget. Fink (1995) defines evaluation as a diligent investigation of a program's characteristics and merits.

Evaluation has also been defined as the process of determining the merits, worth, and value of things/initiatives, and evaluations are the products of that process.

Approaching an evaluation from the viewpoint of a research tradition, there established theories, techniques, and procedures to carry it out.

Purpose

The purpose of an evaluation is often, though not always, determined by the program funder, sometimes in negotiation with the various stakeholders and the evaluator. Its purpose is to provide information on the effectiveness of projects so as to optimize the outcome, efficiency, and quality. Most evaluations serve one or more of the following overlapping functions:

1. They provide information about the ongoing implementation of the initiative so that its progress and strategies can be assessed and midcourse corrections instituted.
2. They build the capacity of the initiative/program participants to design and institutionalize the self-assessment process.
3. They draw some conclusions from judgments about the degree to which the program has achieved its goals.
4. Evaluations support a collaborative process of change that combines creating knowledge with mutual education and mobilization for action.
5. They hold those conducting the initiative/program accountable to the funder, the target area/population stakeholder groups, and society.
6. They contribute to the development of broad knowledge and theory about the implementation and outcomes of the project.
7. They promote public relations and fund-raising capacity.

Strategic Prevention and Intervention Framework

Evaluation activities take place within clearly defined contexts. Monitoring and evaluating anti-bullying programs must be viewed within the context of prevention, intervention, and recovery, a continuum of care. The framework begins with needs assessment. This requires an early engagement/involvement of culturally competent research evaluators. A model for understanding the context for anti-bullying evaluation may be diagrammed (SPIF):

Strategic Prevention/Intervention Framework (SPIF)

3. Strategic Planning

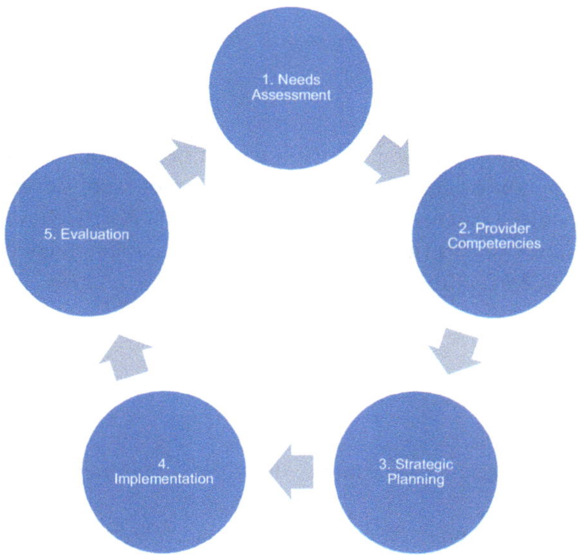

Standards for Program Evaluation

In 1975, the Joint Committee on Standards for Educational Evaluation (JCSEE) was founded as a coalition of major professional associations concerned with the quality of evaluation. The Joint Committee is a private, nonprofit organization that is accredited by the American National Standards Institute. It reviews and updates its published standards every 5 years. It also trains policymakers, evaluators, and educators on the use of the standards and serves as a clearing house on evaluation standard literature (JCSEE 1975). The standards provide guidelines for designing, implementing, assessing, and improving the identified form of evaluation. It is important to note that each of the standards has been placed in one of four fundamental categories to promote educational evaluations that are proper, useful, feasible, and accurate. (http://en.wikipedia.org/wiki/joint_committee_on_standards updated 2017)

Contents

6. References
7. External Links

Joint Committee on Standards for Educational Evaluation (2011).

Guiding Principles for Evaluators

The American Evaluation Association Guiding Principles have been adopted for application in anti-bullying program evaluation. The AEA principles were developed and endorsed in 1994, reviewed and revised in 2004 by the AEA. A full text of the principles is available online at www.eval.org. The following is an abbreviated version. (http://www.eval.org/P/CM/ID/fid=51)

AEA Guiding Principles: Executive Summary

A. *Systematic inquiry:* Evaluators conduct systematic, data-based inquiries about whatever is being evaluated.
B. *Competence:* Evaluators provide competent performance to stakeholders.
C. *Integrity and honesty*: Evaluators ensure the honesty and integrity of the entire evaluation process.
D. *Respect for people*: Evaluators respect the security, dignity, and self-worth of the respondents, program participants, clients, and other stakeholders with whom they interact.
E. *Responsibilities for general and public welfare*: Evaluators articulate and take into account the diversity of interests and values that may be related to the general and public welfare.

The Principles

A. *Systematic inquiry*: Evaluators conduct systematic, data-based inquiries.

   1. To ensure the accuracy and credibility of the evaluative information they produce, evaluators should adhere to the highest technical standards appropriate to the methods they use.
   2. Evaluators should explore with the client the shortcomings and strengths of both the various evaluation questions and the various approaches that might be used for answering those questions.
   3. Evaluators should communicate their methods and approaches accurately and in sufficient detail to allow others to understand, interpret, and critique their work. They should make clear the limitations of an evaluation and its

results. Evaluators should discuss in a contextually appropriate way those values, assumptions, theories, methods, results, and significantly affecting the interpretation of the evaluative findings.

These assessments should be applied to all aspects of the evaluation, from the initial conceptualization to the eventual use of finding.

B. *Competence*: Evaluators provide competent performance to stakeholders.

1. Evaluators should possess (or ensure that the evaluation team possesses) the education, abilities, skills, and experience appropriate to undertake the task proposed in the evaluation.
2. To ensure recognition, accurate interpretation, and respect for diversity evaluators should ensure that the members of the evaluation team collectively demonstrate cultural competence. Cultural competence would be reflected in evaluators seeking awareness of their own culturally based assumptions, their understanding of the worldviews of culturally different participants and stakeholders in the evaluation, and the use of appropriate evaluation strategies and skills in working with culturally different groups. Diversity may be in terms of race, ethnicity, gender, religion, socioeconomics, or other factors pertinent to the evaluation context.
3. Evaluators should practice within the limits of their professional training and competence and should decline to conduct evaluations that fall substantially outside those limits. When declining the commission or request is not feasible or appropriate, evaluators should make clear any significant limitations on the evaluation that might result. Evaluators should make it an effort to gain the competence directly or through the assistance of others who possess the required expertise.
4. Evaluators should continually seek to maintain and improve their competencies, in order to provide the highest level of performance in their evaluations. This continuing professional development might include formal coursework and workshops, self-study, evaluation of one's own practice, and working with other evaluators to learn from their skills and expertise.

C. *Integrity and honesty*: Evaluators display honesty and integrity in their own behavior and attempt to ensure the honesty and integrity of the entire evaluation process.

1. Evaluators should negotiate honestly with clients and relevant stakeholders concerning the costs, tasks to be undertaken, limitations of methodology, scope of results likely to be obtained, and uses of data resulting from a specific evaluation. It is primarily the evaluators responsibility to initiate discussion and clarification of these matters, not the client's.
2. Before accepting an evaluation assignment, evaluators should disclose any roles or relationships that might pose a conflict of interest (or appearance with their role as an evaluator). If they proceed with the evaluation, the conflict(s) should be clearly articulated in reports of the evaluation results.

3. Evaluators should record all changes made in the originally negotiated project plans and the reasons why the changes were made. If those changes would significantly affect the scope and likely results of the evaluation, the evaluator should inform the client and other important stakeholders in a timely fashion (barring good reason to the contrary, before proceeding with further work) of the changes and their likely impact.
4. Evaluators should be explicit about their own, their clients', and other stakeholders' interests and values concerning the conduct and outcomes of an evaluation.
5. Evaluators should not misrepresent their procedures, data, or findings. Within reasonable limits, they should attempt to prevent or correct misuse of their work by others.
6. If evaluators determine that certain procedures or activities are likely to produce misleading evaluative information or conclusions, they have the responsibility to communicate their concerns and the reasons for them. If discussions with the client do not resolve these concerns, the evaluator should decline to conduct the evaluation. If declining the assignment is unfeasible or inappropriate, the evaluator should consult colleagues or relevant stakeholders about other appropriate ways to proceed. (Options include discussions at a higher level, a dissenting cover letter or appendix, or refusal to sign the final document.)
7. Evaluators should disclose all sources of financial support for an evaluation and the source of the request for evaluation.

D. *Respect for people:* Evaluators respect the security, dignity, and self-worth of respondents, program participants, clients, and other evaluation stakeholders.

1. Evaluators should seek a comprehensive understanding of the relevant contextual elements of the evaluation. Contextual factors that may influence the results of a study include geographic location, timing, political and social climate, economic conditions, and other relevant activities in progress at the same time.
2. Evaluators should abide by current professional ethics, standards, and regulations regarding risks, harms, and burdens that might befall those participating in the evaluation and regarding informed consent for participation in evaluation and regarding information participants and clients about the scope and limits of confidentiality.
3. Because of the negative or critical conclusions from an evaluation which must be explicitly stated, evaluations sometimes produce results that harm clients or stakeholder interests. Under this circumstance, evaluators should seek to maximize the benefits and reduce any unnecessary harms that might occur, provided this will not compromise the integrity of the evaluation findings. Evaluators should carefully judge when the benefit of doing the evaluation or in performing certain procedures should be foregone because of the risks or harms. To the extent possible, these issues should be anticipated during the negotiation of the evaluation.
4. Knowing that evaluations may negatively affect the interests of some stakeholders, evaluators should conduct the evaluation and communicate its

results in a way that clearly respects the stakeholders' dignity and self-worth.

5. Where feasible, evaluators should attempt to foster social equity in evaluation, so that those who contribute to the evaluation may benefit in return. Program participants should be informed that their eligibility to receive services does not hinge on their participation in the evaluation.
6. Evaluators have the responsibility to understand and respect differences among participants, such as differences in their culture, religion, gender disability, age, sexual orientation, and ethnicity, and to account for potential implications of these differences when planning, conducting, analyzing, and reporting evaluations.

E. *Responsibilities for general and public welfare*: Evaluators articulate and take into account the diversity of general and public interests and that may be related to the evaluation.

1. When planning and reporting evaluations, evaluators should include relevant perspectives and interests of the full range stakeholders.
2. Evaluators should consider not only the immediate operations and outcomes of whatever is evaluated but also their broad assumptions, implications, and potential side effects.
3. Freedom of information is essential in a democracy. Evaluators should allow all relevant stakeholders access to evaluative information in forms that respect people and honor promises of confidentiality. Evaluators should actively disseminate information to stakeholders as resources allow. Communications that are tailored to a given stakeholder should include all results that may bear on interest of that stakeholder and refer to any other tailored communications to other stakeholders. In all cases, evaluators should strive to present results clearly and simply so that clients and other stakeholders can easily understand the evaluation process and results.
4. Evaluators should maintain a balance between client needs and other needs. Evaluators necessarily have a special relationship with the client who funds or requests the evaluation. By virtue of that relationship, evaluators must strive to meet legitimate client needs whenever feasible and appropriate to do so. However, that relationship can also place evaluators in difficult dilemmas when client interests conflict with other interests or when client interests conflict with the obligation of evaluators for systematic inquiry, competence, integrity, and respect for people. In these cases, evaluators should explicitly identify and discuss the conflicts with the client and relevant stakeholders, resolve them when possible, determine whether continued work on the evaluation is advisable if the conflicts cannot be resolved, and make clear any significant limitations on the evaluation that it may be the case that the conflict is not resolved.
5. Evaluators have obligations that encompass the public interest and good. These obligations are especially important when evaluators are supported by publicly generated funds; but clear threats to the public good should never be ignored in any evaluation. Because the public interest and good rarely the

same as the interest of any particular group (including those of the client), evaluators will usually have to go beyond the analysis of particular stakeholder interests and consider the welfare of society as a whole.

Evaluation Models

There are several program evaluation approaches/models that have been used or can be used for anti-bullying program evaluation. The list includes the following:

- Olweus
- Risk and protective factors
- Disciplinary approach
- Comparison group
- Experimental group
- Social and emotional learning (SEL)
- Logic model
- Meta-analysis
- Ecological approach

While each of the above and the others have merit, there is sufficient evidence in the literature to recommend the logic model as the most effective evaluation model for monitoring and evaluating anti-bullying programs.

Logic Model

In 1998, the W.K. Kellogg Foundation published the W.K. Kellogg Foundation Handbook in response to the growing need for nonprofits to demonstrate the effectiveness of their program activities by initiating and completing outcome-oriented evaluation of projects. The handbook provides a framework for thinking about evaluation as a relevant and useful program tool. It is guided by the belief that evaluation should be supportive and responsive to projects, rather than become an end in itself. The handbook is made up of two distinct parts. Part one reviews the contextual factors that have led to an imbalance in how human service evaluation is defined and conducted and includes recommendations for creating a better balance between proving that programs work and improving how the word and why. Part two provides a description of various components of project-level evaluation that can assist project staff in addressing a broad array of important questions about the project. It should be noted here that W.K. Kellogg Foundation was established in 1930 "to help people help themselves through the practical application of knowledge and resources to improve the quality of life and that of future generations" (www.wkkf.org).

What Is Logic Model?

According to W.K. Kellogg Foundation Evaluation Handbook (1998, p 35), "A Program Logic Model is a picture of how your program works -- the theory and assumptions underlying the program. …This model provides a road map of your program, highlighting how it is expected to work, what activities need to come before others, and how desired outcomes are achieved." The logic model is a beneficial evaluation tool that facilitates effective program planning, implementation, and evaluation. Experience supports the notion that effective program evaluation does more than collect, analyze, and provide data. It makes it possible for program staff and stakeholders to gather and use information, to learn continually about, and to improve programs. The logic model is a learning and management tool that can be used throughout a program's life. There is overwhelming evidence that using the logic model as an evaluation tool, especially for Kellogg Foundation funded projects, has resulted in effective programming and offers greater learning opportunities, better documentation of outcomes, and shared knowledge about what works and why, and many evaluation experts have concluded that the use of the logic model is an effective way to ensure program success. As Ricardo Millert, Director of WKKF Evaluation Unit, has noted, "The bane of evaluation is a poorly designed program."

Why Use a Logic Model?

Three important reasons for using the logic model can be summarized from the literature:

1. In program design and planning, the logic model serves as a planning tool to develop program strategy and enhance your ability to clearly explain and illustrate program concepts and approach for key stakeholders, including funders. It can help craft structure and organization for program design and build in self-evaluation based on shared understanding of what it is to take place.
2. In program implementation, the logic model forms the core of a focused management plan that helps you identify and collect the data needed to monitor and improve programming using the logic model during program implementation, and management requires you to focus energies on achieving and documenting results. It helps to consider and prioritize the program aspects most critical for tracking and reporting and make adjustments as necessary.
3. For program evaluation and strategic reporting, the logic model provides periodic feedback to program managers. This allows program managers to make the necessary adjustments toward achieving their goals. It also allows them to mobilize resources for the sustainability of their programs. The figure below shows how to read a logic model (Wholey et al. 1994; Bailey et al. 1998).

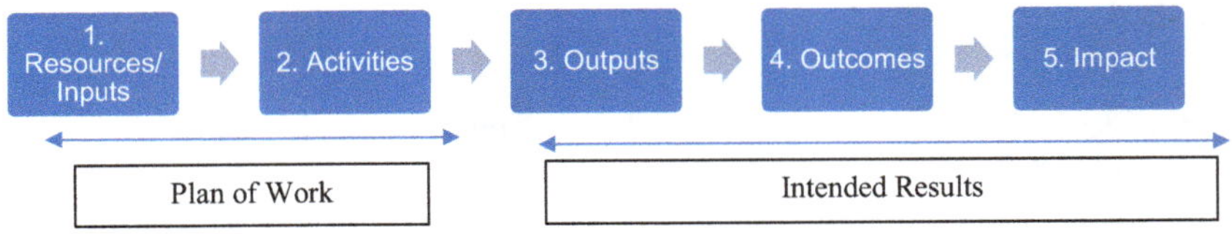

1. Resources/inputs: Certain resources are needed to operate program. These resources are usually funds, staff, and facilities.
2. Activities: Resources are used to accomplish planned activities.
3. Outputs: These are products or severe that are intended; these are contingent on accomplishing planned activities in 2.
4. Outcomes: Ideally planned activities lead to intended outcomes/results, program participants benefit.
5. Impact: Certain changes in organizations, communities, or systems, and/or behaviors are expected to occur.

It is important to note hear that, in practice, most logic models are more complex and fall into one of three categories: the theory approach model (conceptual), outcome approach model, or activities approach model (applied)—or a blend of several types. It is not unusual for a program to use all three types of logic models for different purposes. For the purpose of anti-bullying program evaluation, all three types are highly recommended.

Program Evaluation Reporting

It is important for the program administrators and evaluation researchers to develop effective communication strategies for disseminating evaluation research findings on programs for a broad range of audiences, including stakeholders, funders, school constituencies, policymakers, students, parents, law enforcement groups, members of the faith-based communities, etc.

Dissemination Strategies

Traditionally, the dissemination of program outcomes has been for the most part limited to the use of the media, especially the print media. An effective dissemination strategy must consider the use of various communication channels. Such a dissemination strategy may be diagrammed as follows:

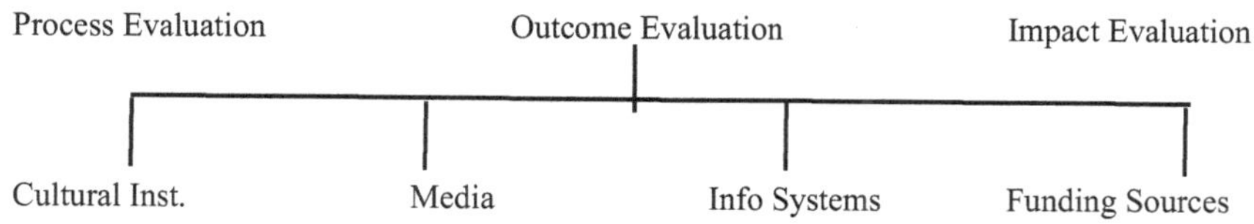

• Schools • Post Secondary Education • Museums • Spirituality • Music • Visual and Performing Arts • Libraries and Archives	• Print • Television • Radio • Film • Video • Tapes	• Computer (software) • Computer (on-line networks) • Publishers	• Progress Reports • Annual Reports

Source: Adopted from American Health Coalition, Inc. training manual, 2017

References

Bailey, Z., Phillips, C., & James, M. (1998). *Decoding program logic models*. Chicago IL: Annual Meeting of the American Evaluation Association.

Educational Evaluation. (1975). Joint Committee Standards for Educational Evaluation Report.

Fink, A. (1995). A Galileo Analysis of Organizational Climate. New York: Wiley & Sons Publishing.

Joint Committee on Standards for Educational Evaluation. (2017). Retrieved from https://en.wikipedia.org/wiki/Joint_Committee_on_Standards_for_Educational_Evaluation

Joint Committee on Standards for Educational Evaluation. (2011). *The Program Evaluation Standards*. Newbury Park, CA: Sage Publications.

Ross, P. H., Ellipse, M. W., & Freeman, H. E. (2004). Evaluation: A systematic approach. 7th ed. Chicago, IL: University of Chicago Press.

Kellogg Foundation, W. K. (1998). *Logic Model Development Guide*. Battle Creek, MI: Kellogg Foundation.

Wholey, J. S., Harry, H. P., & Newcomer, K. E. (1994). *Handbook of practical program evaluation*. San Francisco: Jossey-Bass.

Index

J. U'Mofe Gordon (ed.), *Bullying Prevention and Intervention at School*,
https://doi.org/10.1007/978-3-319-95414-1

MIX
Papier | Fördert
gute Waldnutzung
FSC® C083411

Kolibri 360 GmbH
Ferdinand-Jühlke-Straße 7
99095 Erfurt, Deutschland
produktsicherheit@kolibri360.de